THE
NEW BIBLE
CURE
FOR HEART
DISEASE

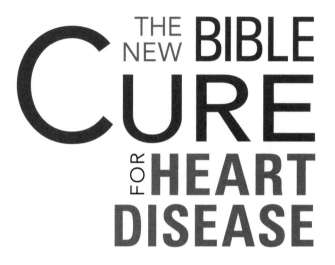

THE NEW BIBLE CURE FOR HEART DISEASE

DON COLBERT, MD

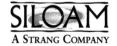

SILOAM

A STRANG COMPANY

Most STRANG COMMUNICATIONS BOOK GROUP products are available at special quantity discounts for bulk purchase for sales promotions, premiums, fund-raising, and educational needs. For details, write Strang Communications Book Group, 600 Rinehart Road, Lake Mary, Florida 32746, or telephone (407) 333-0600.

THE NEW BIBLE CURE FOR HEART DISEASE by Don Colbert, MD
Published by Siloam, a Strang Company
600 Rinehart Road
Lake Mary, Florida 32746
www.strangbookgroup.com

Unless otherwise noted, all Scripture quotations are from the Holy Bible, New Living Translation, copyright © 1996, 2004. Used by permission of Tyndale House Publishers, Inc., Wheaton, IL 60189. All rights reserved.

Scripture quotations marked KJV are from the King James Version of the Bible.

Cover design by Amanda Potter; Design Director: Bill Johnson

Library of Congress Cataloging in Publication:
Colbert, Don.
  The new bible cure for heart disease / by Don Colbert.
      p. cm.
  Includes bibliographical references.
  ISBN 978-1-59979-869-1
  1. Heart--Diseases--Prevention--Religious aspects. 2. Healing--Religious aspects. I. Title.

RC682.C59 2010
616.1'205--dc22

2010018823

10 11 12 13 14 — 9 8 7 6 5 4 3 2 1
Printed in the United States of America

CONTENTS

A NEW BIBLE CURE WITH NEW HOPE FOR YOUR HEART

HOPE BEATS THE statistics and will help you overcome the threat of cardiovascular disease. In the United States, over 800,000 people a year die from disease related to the cardiovascular system. Nearly another 150,000 die from strokes, which are the equivalent of a "heart attack of the brain." While the good news is that these numbers are on the decrease, the bad news is that cardiovascular disease is still the leading cause of death in the United States. Instead of becoming one of these statistics, you can take positive steps naturally and spiritually to beat heart disease. The risk of heart attacks can still be greatly lessened through dietary and lifestyle changes.[1]

In fact, cardiovascular disease is one of the most treatable and preventable of all afflictions, despite the fact that it causes *more than one in three of all deaths* in the United States every year.[2] That means you can fight back, overcome, and win the battle. Through lifestyle changes, good nutrition, prayer, and Scripture reading, you can respond in confident hope to this disease.

The initial symptoms and warning signs of heart disease are not a death sentence, but they are a life warning. Change is required. Positive steps must be taken. The way you live and eat cannot remain the same if you want to have a healthy and strong heart. Take courage, and be hopeful. You and God will prevail as you learn about the Bible cure for cardiovascular disease.

Originally published as *The Bible Cure for Heart Disease* in 1999, *The New Bible Cure for Heart Disease* has been revised and updated with the latest medical research on this disease. If you compare it side by side with the previous edition, you'll see that it's also larger, allowing me to expand greatly upon the information provided in the previous edition and provide you with a deeper understanding of what you face and how to overcome it.

Unchanged from the previous edition are the timeless, life-changing, and healing scriptures throughout this book that will strengthen and encourage your spirit and soul. The proven principles, truths, and guidelines in these passages anchor the practical and medical insights also contained in this book. They will effectively focus your prayers, thoughts, and actions so you can step into God's plan of divine health for you—a plan that includes victory over heart disease.

Another change since the original *The Bible Cure for Heart Disease* was published is that I've released *The Seven Pillars of Health*. I encourage you to read it because the principles of health it contains are the foundation to healthy living that will affect all areas of your life. It sets the stage for everything you will ever read in any other book I've published—including this one.

I pray that these spiritual and practical suggestions for health, nutrition, and fitness will bring wholeness to your life, increase your spiritual understanding, and strengthen and prolong your ability to worship and serve God.

—DR. DON COLBERT

A **BIBLE CURE** Prayer for You

Heavenly Father, open my eyes to the natural and spiritual
ways I can prevent and overcome cardiovascular disease.
Give me the insight to apply all I learn with great wisdom.
And grant me Your abiding peace, freeing me from all
fear, anxiety, and worry as I trust in Your sovereign will.
In the name of the Healer, Jesus of Nazareth, amen.

HOPE TO BEAT THE STATISTICS FOR HEART DISEASE

H AVE YOU EVER considered the marvelous design and operation of your cardiovascular system? It's the body's amazing superhighway. The large arteries within it are much like interstate expressways, and the smaller arteries are like streets and side streets. The primary function of the circulatory system is to deliver oxygen and nutrients to all the cells in your body and to remove cellular debris and waste.

Each day your heart beats approximately 100,000 times pushing about 2,000 gallons of blood through the 60,000 miles of blood vessels in your body, which include arteries, veins, and capillaries. Despite this incredible distance, blood circulates throughout your entire system about once a minute. Thus your heart will beat over 2.5 billion times if you live an average lifespan, and it will pump over 50 billion gallons of blood.[1] This superhighway system is truly wonderful.

Wouldn't it be a good idea to keep this blood vessel superhighway free of traffic jams?

BUILDING A DEADLY BACKUP?

Yes, we might think of heart problems in terms of traffic flow— and a traffic jam. The worst contributor to a potentially deadly backup is a condition called *atherosclerosis*, which attacks the heart's blood vessels. The arteries that supply the heart with blood and nourishment are the coronary arteries. These are the most stressed arteries of the body because they're squeezed flat from the pumping action of the heart.

Atherosclerosis is the hardening of these arteries most commonly due to excessive amounts of plaque. This plaque contains cholesterol, calcium, white blood cells, collagen, elastin, platelets, and other materials. You could compare plaque to a buildup of debris in a pipe. As the plaque builds up in the arteries, blood flow is eventually decreased to vital organs, including the heart and brain. This buildup can lead to an interruption of blood flow to an artery in the brain, which causes a stroke. When blood flow is interrupted in a coronary artery, a heart attack occurs.

FREEING UP THE TRAFFIC

If atherosclerosis is the cause of a traffic jam in the blood flow, you'll be happy to know that forces are at work in your body to free up the traffic jam. I can explain this best by breaking the process into two parts: (1) the problem of free radicals, and (2) the problem of inflammation, which I'll discuss in the next chapter.

The problem: oxidative stress

A *free radical* isn't a terrorist trying to bomb our embassy; rather, it's a defective molecule that sends out molecular shrapnel, damaging the coronary arteries and other cells in our bodies. To envision this problem, think about the oxidation process. Burn wood in a fireplace, and smoke is a by-product. Likewise, when you metabolize food into energy, oxygen oxidizes (or burns) the food in order to produce energy. This process does not create smoke like burning wood in a fireplace, but it does produce dangerous by-products known as free radicals. These are molecules that have electrons roaming free to do damage in other cells. The by-products of oxidation are called free radicals. Isn't it ironic that breathing oxygen is critical for life and that oxygen usage by the cells is our bodies' greatest source of free radicals?

With regard to heart disease, the problem is that free radicals wreak havoc on the linings of arteries. You see, the lining of the coronary arteries is comprised of very sensitive cells that can easily sustain damage by free radicals produced from oxygen free radicals, cigarette smoke, hypertension, excessive stress, high cholesterol, high lipoprotein(a), elevated homocysteine, and other risk factors. Oxidation is a normal biochemical process in the body. However, sometimes excessive amounts of free radicals are produced, or we have inadequate antioxidant protection. This oxidative stress can damage healthy cells and tissues, including the lining of the arteries or endothelium. When LDL cholesterol is oxidized, it is especially damaging to the arterial lining and is associated with plaque formation.

So, free radicals are the enemies of our blood vessels and of our bodies' cells in general. Some estimates calculate that the cells in our bodies may sustain over 10,000 hits from free radicals each day, especially if we have inadequate antioxidants.

> Don't you realize that all of you together are the
> temple of God and that the Spirit of God lives in you?
> God will destroy anyone who destroys this temple.
> For God's temple is holy, and you are that temple.
> —1 CORINTHIANS 3:16–17

The solution: antioxidants

God's Bible cure in winning the battle against heart disease includes a powerful weapon against free radicals—*antioxidants.* They're amazing substances that slow oxidation and block or repair free-radical reactions in our bodies.

The heart is the hardest-working organ in the body. Since the coronary arteries sustain more wear and tear than other arteries, they also need to be constantly repaired. Antioxidants are extremely important in preventing heart disease due to their blocking and repairing functions.

Millions of microscopic cracks and damaged areas may occur inside the artery walls from oxidative damage. When the body does not have adequate amounts of antioxidants, especially glutathione and vitamins C and E, in order to repair the lining of damaged blood vessels, it will be more prone to forming plaque in the arteries. This, along with chronic inflammation, forms fatty streaks in the blood vessels and leads to plaque formation. However, adequate amounts of antioxidants such as gluthathione, vitamins C and E, bioflavonoids, pine bark and grape seed extract, resveratrol, pomegranate juice, and berries such as blueberries, blackberries, raspberries, and strawberries may help prevent these cracks from occurring in the first place. (See appendix.)

Picture it this way: Imagine repairing a house after a tornado has partially damaged the roof and damaged walls. If you didn't have the money to repair the roof and walls properly, and you merely patched them with the inexpensive materials at hand, the next storm might well destroy your dwelling for good.

Likewise, if you have inadequate antioxidants in your diet and you are damaging your blood vessels with smoking, high blood pressure, or a fatty diet, areas of your blood vessels will usually become chronically inflamed and attract monocytes (white blood cells), which are transformed into macrophages, another type of white blood cell. These macrophages are super garbage collectors that gobble up oxidized cholesterol and cellular debris and eventually form fatty streaks and later fatty plaque. However, antioxidant vitamins help to prevent or repair the lining of the blood vessels that are damaged and halt or diminish the destructive inflammatory response. Without adequate antioxidants, more plaque is formed. If this continues over decades, the fatty plaque builds up in your blood vessels, creating atherosclerosis, which can eventually lead to a heart attack. This certainly isn't God's will for you!

> Dear friend, I hope all is well with you and that you are as healthy in body as you are strong in spirit.
> —3 JOHN 2

For a healthy heart, don't forget your citrus fruit and vitamin C. Vitamin C is a very important antioxidant for repairing damage to the coronary arteries. It helps to increase the production of collagen and elastin, both of which add stability to our blood vessels. Collagen produced without vitamin C is weaker and causes blood vessels to become fragile. Scurvy results from an extremely depleted supply of vitamin C reserves in the body. This condition causes a gradual breakdown of collagen, leading to a breakdown in blood vessels, resulting in internal hemorrhaging.

In chapter 3, I'll give you my specific recommendations for combating my top twenty-four heart attack risk factors through diet and nutritional supplements.

A **BIBLE CURE** Health Fact

While many animals can create their own vitamin C, people cannot. We must replenish it daily through our diet. Unfortunately, much of our food is so processed that very little vitamin C remains in our foods. Citrus fruit is a major source of vitamin C, but while most of us may have enough vitamin C to prevent scurvy, we don't have enough to win the war against arteriosclerosis.

LIVING WITH FAITH AND HOPE

When I originally published this book in 1999, the American Heart Association (AHA) reported that one in two deaths was related to heart disease. However, according to 2010 AHA statistics, just over one in three deaths in the United States are now related to cardiovascular disease (CVD), a category of illnesses that includes high blood pressure, coronary heart disease, heart attack, angina, heart failure, and stroke.[2] This means that the number of CVD-related deaths in the United States is declining. In fact, the AHA reports that from 1996 to 2006 the death rate from CVD declined by 29 percent.[3]

While the trends reflected by these statistics are encouraging, we can also be optimistic because heart disease is one of the most preventable of all degenerative diseases. Furthermore, we can take great hope in the reality that God is our healer (Exod. 15:26). Nutrition and lifestyle changes are the cornerstones in keeping it at bay. Prayer is a great resource in building our hope and opening our lives up to God's healing power.

The major contributors to heart disease are unhealthy diet, lack of exercise, obesity (especially belly fat), smoking, hypertension, and elevated cholesterol. Clearly, these six factors are within our control. And you can make a decision to put your faith and trust in God's Spirit to help you implement the steps you need to take to eat healthily, exercise, lose belly fat or maintain a healthy weight, stop smoking, and lower your blood pressure and cholesterol.

Yes, there is hope for this amazing, hardworking superhighway vascular system in your body. It can keep the nutrients flowing for years and years with no roadblocks or breakdowns. So I encourage you to live each day in faith and hope, while taking some important preventive steps right away. Make this your hope:

> Let all that I am wait quietly before God,
>   for my hope is in him.
> He alone is my rock and my salvation,
>   my fortress where I will not be shaken.
>
> —PSALM 62:5–6

In this book, you will learn about the factors that put you at risk and what to do about them. Make a decision now to implement what you learn.

A **BIBLE CURE** Health Fact

A simple warning sign of heart disease is a diagonal crease in the earlobes. If you have creases in the earlobes, there is a strong probability you have significant atherosclerosis in your coronary arteries.[4] Also, according to a Harvard study, men who are losing the hair on the crown of their heads have up to a 34 percent greater risk of having cardiovascular problems.[5]

A **BIBLE CURE** Prayer for You

Heavenly Father, I know that I have some important choices to make. I can put myself at greater risk for a heart attack, or I can take steps now to reduce my risk. You have put some powerful resources and information in my hands for living a healthier life. Help me to use what I know and implement positive steps in both the natural and spiritual realms to prevent heart disease. Amen.

A **BIBLE CURE** Prescription
What Do You Think?

What antioxidants can you include in your diet and supplements to quench free radicals?

_____ Citrus fruits

_____ Pomegranate juice

_____ Berries

_____ Vitamin C

_____ Bioflavonoids

_____ Pine bark and grape seed extract

_____ Vitamin E

_____ Glutathione-boosting supplements

_____ Resveratrol

INFLAMMATION: THE ROOT CAUSE OF HEART DISEASE

EART DISEASE IS hidden in more than half of all adults over the age of thirty-five. That is more than half of your family and friends. Many think that because their cholesterol is normal, they are protected against heart disease, but science is finding that keeping our arteries healthy is about much more than just cholesterol levels. About half of the people who have heart attacks have normal cholesterol levels. The root cause of heart disease is not high cholesterol but *inflammation*.

THE GOOD AND BAD OF INFLAMMATION

Inflammation actually means "fire inside," because inflamed areas often feel like they are burning from within. Inflammation is the redness, swelling, pain, and heat that occur in an area of the body as a consequence of infection, injury, or a foreign object such as a splinter. For example, if you have strep tonsillitis, your tonsils are infected with a strep bacterium, and they are generally swollen, red, and very painful. A sprained ankle is simply inflammation in the ankle, and the ankle is usually red, swollen, painful, and warm. A splinter that is embedded in your skin may eventually form an abscess or boil that is red, swollen, warm, and painful.

This is the good side of inflammation—the healing side. Acute inflammation is meant to save your life or speed up healing by sending white blood cells to the area that is inflamed in order to fight the infection, splint the injury, or wall off the inflammation, which occurs in an abscess.

Acute inflammation on the molecular level is similar to a war. First, your immune system recognizes an invader such as an infection or injury and sends troops in the form of white blood cells to the area being attacked by using chemical signals. Similar to troops going into battle, these white blood cells receive instructions to defend the area that is injured or under attack. The white blood cells then swarm the injured area and secrete different chemical "weapons" in order to eradicate the infection. Now you are beginning to visualize the good side of inflammation—its role in fighting invaders such as bacteria and viruses and eliminating them from the body.

Now let's look at the dark side of inflammation. Realize that the same inflammation that can save your life in the short term can also kill you if inflammation becomes chronic. Your coronary arteries are composed of three layers. Most think of arteries and blood vessels as simple, supple tubes, but in reality they are dynamic muscular structures that expand and contract to aid in circulation and keep blood pressure stable. The outer layer is the *adventitia*. The middle layer is made of smooth muscle, which enables the arteries to dilate and constrict and is called the *medial layer*. The inner layer, called the *intima* or *endothelium*, is smooth like Teflon and is a very thin layer only one cell thick.

As we age, areas of the smooth and slick endothelium lining of the arteries, which is similar to Teflon, eventually become injured by various factors, including high blood pressure, oxidation of

LDL cholesterol, cigarette smoke, free radicals, elevated homocysteine levels, elevated CRP levels, elevated blood sugar and insulin levels, bad fats, poor diet, toxic chemicals and metals, etc. These single or combined *insults* to areas of the coronary arteries kindle inflammation, which is what leads to atherosclerosis.

The presence of chemicals associated with inflammation called *cytokines* causes the inner layer of the arteries to become more like Velcro rather than Teflon. In areas of the coronary arteries that have been damaged by high blood pressure, cigarette smoke, or other factors, the presence of these inflammatory cytokines attracts a type of white blood cell called *monocytes*.

These monocytes eventually transform into *macrophages*, which are even more powerful than the monocytes. Macrophages gobble up dead cells as well as cellular garbage, including oxidized cholesterol. (Oxidized cholesterol is the most damaging type of cholesterol and will be discussed later on.) These macrophages eat and eat, literally stuffing themselves with oxidized cholesterol and cellular garbage as they continue to grow larger and larger.

When chronic inflammation is present, the macrophages continue to eat and may grow so large that they appear like foam and are called *foam cells*. As inflammation continues, the macrophages continue to eat until they eventually "eat themselves to death." When they die, their contents are spilled in the arterial wall and appear as a fatty yellow streak inside the artery. Because of this, researchers are beginning to realize treating heart disease may be more about controlling chronic inflammation than about simply lowering cholesterol levels in the bloodstream. Because of this, many new risk factors for cardiovascular disease are being identified and are being addressed—and these will be discussed in the next chapter.

However, if you quench the fire of inflammation, your arteries will attempt to heal themselves by forming a fibrous cap. A fibrous cap is called *stable plaque* and is much less likely to rupture than unstable plaque. The fibrous cap consists of scar tissue and will typically remain stable as long as the inflammation is controlled. In addition to this, there is good evidence that by quenching chronic inflammation and modifying certain risk factors, we will be able to stabilize the plaque and sometimes actually reverse atherosclerosis.

If inflammation is not stopped and chronic inflammation continues unabated, the fatty streak will continue to grow into fatty plaque. As these foam cells die and release their fatty contents, the plaque forms a fatty core, which is a soft yellow liquid similar in consistency to liquid margarine. As this process continues unabated, the fatty core will keep expanding as more and more macrophages continue to eat and eat the oxidized cholesterol and cellular garbage and continue to grow and eventually die. Ultimately, if this inflammatory process is not stopped, your body's own immune system may actually kill you through mechanisms involving chronic inflammation.

Chronic inflammation may eventually cause the fibrous cap to rupture, similar to popping a large pimple. The fatty liquid margarine–like material will ooze out of the plaque. Immediately, platelets will stick to the oozing fatty material like a swarm of flies to fly paper, and a blood clot forms. As this blood clot blocks the flow of blood, it cuts off vital oxygen and nutrients and causes a heart attack or stroke, depending on which artery it occurs in. If it occurs in a coronary artery, a heart attack occurs. If it occurs in a cerebral or carotid artery, a stroke occurs. Approximately 80 percent of heart attacks are from ruptured plaque.[1]

If you are lucky enough to reach the hospital in time, the doctor will quickly give you a clot-busting drug or insert a stent to open the blocked artery. A clot-busting drug will dissolve the clot, allowing the blood to flow again to the heart, but it does not dissolve the plaque. Individuals typically do not accumulate plaque in just one or two areas but in dozens of areas. Each area may rupture, and just one rupture can cause a heart attack. Also, a plaque buildup may cause only a 20 percent blockage, but even that small an area of plaque can still rupture and cause a heart attack.

A **BIBLE CURE** Health Fact

Plaque in the coronary artery usually starts developing in our teens. During the Korean War when soldiers died in battle at an average age of twenty-two, they were autopsied, and three-quarters of them had plaque in their coronary arteries, many of whom had advanced atherosclerotic plaque. A study was done on 3,000 bodies age fourteen to thirty-five who were autopsied after death from auto accident, homicide, or suicide. Of those autopsied, 20 to 25 percent had a major lesion in their coronary arteries.[2]

This is the dark side of inflammation, which is at the root of most heart disease. There is, however, very good news: we can quench the fires of chronic inflammation. Consuming a diet that is anti-inflammatory as well as taking specific antioxidants and nutrients and modifying cardiovascular risk factors can effectively quench the fires of inflammation and prevent—and in many cases even reverse—cardiovascular disease.

START BY TESTING YOUR CRP LEVEL

Current research is finding that LDL and total cholesterol levels alone are not the best indicators of whether or not heart attacks will happen. Approximately half the time, cardiac arrest is the first symptom of cardiovascular disease someone will experience, and doctors estimate that about 50 percent of those with normal cholesterol levels will still have heart attacks or strokes. While those with high LDL and total cholesterol are three times more likely than those with low levels to experience heart attacks or strokes, there are far too many with "acceptable" levels who have heart attacks every day.[3] Approximately half the patients who suffer heart attacks have normal cholesterol levels. Many individuals think that because their cholesterol is normal or low, they are protected against cardiovascular disease. How wrong they are. Hosea 4:6 says, "My people are destroyed for lack of knowledge" (KJV).

Chronic inflammation can be detected by a simple blood test. We now have a blood test that measures the level of C-reactive protein (CRP) that detects the chronic inflammation that contributes to coronary artery disease.[4] C-reactive protein is both a marker and a promoter of inflammation in the body. Chronically elevated CRP blood levels are indicative that you have systemic inflammation. This is why in 2003 the American Heart Association (AHA) and the Centers for Disease Control and Prevention (CDC) started recommending adding CRP blood tests to regular annual checkups. (For more on tests for cardiovascular risk, see chapter 6.)

Healthy lifestyle choices like the anti-inflammatory diet and other recommendations I will be explaining later in this book are the best way to lower risk factors that lead to arterial inflammation. Where most doctors will recommend statin drugs as a solution, I would caution you before following that course. Study after study has shown that lifestyle changes, if combined with a healthy diet and proper nutritional supplements, can have the same or better results than taking a daily statin drug, and without the side effects.

For example, a few years ago a clinical study, the Jupiter study, was done to determine if the statin drug Crestor would decrease the risk of heart attack and stroke if given to patients with moderate LDL cholesterol levels and elevated levels of C-reactive protein. Crestor did indeed significantly decrease heart attack and stroke incidents—there was a 43 percent reduction in different types of vascular disease after less than two years—but there was still a significant number of heart attacks and strokes in the people whose LDL cholesterol was reduced to very low levels. Crestor—which is primarily designed to lower LDL levels—did also decrease CRP by 37 percent, which was good, but many of the patients still had a CRP level that was too high.[5]

In other words, Crestor is able to reduce LDL cholesterol to very low levels, but lowering LDL levels is usually simply not enough and usually does not adequately quench the fire of inflammation. And even though it lowered CRP, many times it did not lower it enough. There are also many other risk factors that must be addressed (as we will discuss in the next chapter).

A **BIBLE CURE** *Health Fact*

The Women's Health Study of apparently healthy postmenopausal women found women with the highest CRP levels had five times the risk of developing cardiovascular disease and seven times the risk of heart attack or stroke compared to women with the lowest CRP levels.[6]

The bottom line is that researchers are finding many more factors that can *independently* lead to cardiovascular disease than just those that deal with lowering LDL and overall cholesterol levels, the very thing addressed by most statin drugs. Even drugs that address the trifecta of high LDL, low HDL, and high triglycerides are not enough to handle the multitude of risk factors that can cause heart disease.

While this gives a much more complicated picture of heart disease than we have had in the past, the good news is twofold: first is that cardiovascular disease is totally preventable if we take the proper precautions to quench chronic inflammation, and second, apply the keys to a healthy lifestyle through the anti-inflammatory diet; regular exercise; eliminating smoking, secondhand smoke, and other pollutants; lowering blood pressure; living in God's peace and joy; and taking natural supplements that God has readily provided for us.

THE IMPORTANCE OF
AN ANTI-INFLAMMATORY DIET

What you eat is the single most important factor in quenching inflammation, and the healthiest way to eat is still sticking to what God has naturally provided for us on the earth. The Mediterranean diet is an excellent anti-inflammatory diet, and I discuss it in detail in my book *What Would Jesus Eat?* Also, belly fat is a major cause of chronic inflammation, and I also discuss an anti-inflammatory diet to lose belly fat in my book *Dr. Colbert's "I Can Do This" Diet.* God created our bodies, and He knows how they have been designed to function best. Thus the more processed and packaged a food—the less natural it is—the less healthy and usually the more inflammatory it is as well. This is why many poor countries that don't have half the health care system we have in the United States still have a significantly lower incidence of heart disease because they also don't have half the processed, packaged, and inflammatory foods that we do. These products tend to be full of preservatives, saturated and trans fats, sodium, sugar, high-glycemic carbohydrates, and other things that—though they taste good—in the long run are inflammatory and very detrimental to our vascular health. However, there are some changes you can make to what you eat that can make all the difference in the world to when—and if—you will face a cardiovascular incident.

The first is to limit your fat consumption. Take a dramatic step here as soon as possible! Reduce your intake of the saturated fats found in red meat, pork (especially bacon), processed meats (such as bacon, sausage, bologna, salami, pepperoni), whole milk, cheese, butter, ice cream, fried foods, and chicken skins.

Even more dangerous to the health of your heart than saturated fats are *trans fats*. These are found in margarine, many processed peanut butters, many processed foods, pastries, cookies, doughnuts, and cake icing—they can even be found in many so-called "health products." I recommend limiting the amount of fat consumed to less than 30 percent of daily calories, decreasing saturated fats to 7 percent or less of your total calories, and avoiding trans fats altogether.

The fats we consume should be coming from *good* fat sources rather than saturated or trans fat sources. The good fats you should consume are the *omega-3 fatty acids*, which include flaxseed oil and seeds; raw nuts such as almonds, pecans, and macadamia nuts; green leafy vegetables; and cold saltwater fish such as wild salmon, tongol tuna, sardines, and anchovies. In general, the more omega-3 oils that individuals eat, the less coronary artery disease they experience.

Substituting extra-virgin olive oil for butter and cream decreases your risk of developing atherosclerosis. This is no doubt one of the reasons why the Mediterranean diet, or a diet high in olive oil and low in saturated fats, is associated with a lower risk of heart disease. Other healthy monounsaturated fats include avocados, macadamia nuts, almonds, and olives. Also realize that most Americans consume way too many polyunsaturated fats or omega-6 fats. These include sunflower oil, safflower oil, cottonseed oil, soybean oil, corn oil, and most other vegetable oils. These oils are very inflammatory and are found in many salad dressings, sauces, processed foods, restaurant foods, and fast foods. Below is how this type of diet typically looks.

THE MEDITERRANEAN DIET

Most of the following ingredients, which are a part of the Mediterranean diet, are consumed daily. (For a more detailed description of this diet than what follows, refer to my previous books *Eat This and Live*, *Dr. Colbert's "I Can Do This" Diet*, and *What Would Jesus Eat?*)

- *Olive oil* replaces most fats, oils, butter, and margarine. It is used in salads as well as for cooking. Extra-virgin olive oil raises levels of the good cholesterol (HDL) and strengthens the immune system.

- *Bread.* Consumed daily and prepared as whole-grain, dark, chewy, crusty loaves. Eat whole-grain breads and avoid white processed bread. I prefer Ezekiel 4:9 bread or sprouted breads.

- *Whole-grain pasta, brown or wild rice, couscous, bulgur, potatoes.* Often served with fresh vegetables and herbs sautéed in olive oil. Occasionally served with small quantities of lean beef.

- *Grains.* Consumed regularly, such as wheat bran (½ cup, five to seven times weekly); alternate with a cereal such as All Bran, Fiber One, or Bran Buds (½ cup) or other cereals that contain oats or oat bran (⅓ cup).

- *Fruit*, preferably raw, two to three pieces daily; *and nuts*, especially pecans, almonds, and macadamia nuts, at least ten per day.

- *Beans.* Include pintos, great northern, navy, and kidney beans. Beans and lentil soups are very popular (prepared with a small amount of olive oil). Have at least ½ cup of beans, three to four times weekly.

- *Vegetables.* Dark green variety, especially in salads. Start lunch and dinner with a large, colorful salad with romaine lettuce, spinach, or other healthy greens, and use extra-virgin olive oil and vinegar. Eat at least one serving of the following daily: cabbage, broccoli, cauliflower, turnip greens, mustard greens, carrots, spinach, or sweet potatoes.

- *Cheese and yogurt.* Small amounts of low-fat cheese may be grated on soups or meals. Use the reduced-fat varieties. (The fat-free cheeses often taste like rubber.) I prefer feta, provolone, and mozzarella low-fat cheeses. The best yogurt is plain and fat free or low fat but not frozen and with fruit. Add your own fruit to the yogurt. I prefer nonfat Greek yogurt with fruit.

Include the following foods in your diet only a few times weekly:

- *Fish.* The healthiest fish are cold-water varieties such as wild salmon, tongol tuna, and sardines. These are high in omega-3 fatty acids.

- *Poultry.* Eaten two to three times weekly. Choose white breast meat with the skin removed.

- *Eggs.* Eaten only in small amounts (two to three per week).

- *Red meat.* Only rarely, on an average of three times a month. Use only lean cuts with the fat trimmed, and free range or organic is preferred. Use in small amounts as an additive to spice up soup or pasta. (Note: the severe restriction of red meat in the Mediterranean diet is a radical departure from the American diet, but it is a major contributor to the low rates of cancer and heart disease found in these countries.) I also recommend less than 18 ounces of red meat a week to reduce the risk of prostate cancer.

To make sure you are getting all the nutrition that you need, you will also want to add the proper dietary supplements to your daily intake. Proper nutrition combined with exercise and coping with stress are your strongest allies against the threats of cardiovascular disease.

However, it is also good that you understand why these will help you as well as what other, smaller things you should do to address heart health. With that in mind, we will look at the twenty-four most significant risk factors for cardiovascular disease in the next chapter. While these can seem overwhelming,

I want you to remember that God has provided hope for us against this giant of a killer. Like David, we can be assured of God's help if we will heed the wisdom of His Bible cure.

A **BIBLE CURE** Prayer for You

Almighty God, thank You for my cardiovascular system. Speak Your healing words to my heart. Help me to stay on track in my diet so that my food will bring nourishment and healing. Thank You, Lord, for healing me. Amen.

A **BIBLE CURE** Prescription
Healthy First Steps

You can begin to find hope for a healthy vascular system by taking these simple first steps today. Check off the ones you are now taking, and underline the ones you need to start immediately.

- ❏ Limit bad fats (saturated and polyunsaturated), and avoid all trans fats.

- ❏ Follow the Mediterranean diet.

- ❏ Address your stress, and use promises from God's Word to cope with stress.

- ❏ Stop smoking.

- ❏ Exercise regularly.

- ❏ Consult your physician or a nutritional doctor.

- ❏ Pray for God's guidance and healing.

DR. COLBERT'S TOP RISK FACTORS OF CARDIOVASCULAR DISEASE—AND HOW TO BEAT THEM WITH NUTRITION

F IFTY YEARS FROM now, health care professionals may look back at our time and scratch their heads, wondering how so many died of cardiovascular (CV) disease when there were so many proven methods for detecting and correcting its dangers. After all, the causes of heart disease and stroke are becoming clearer each day. Yet at the same time millions still have the ticking time bomb of atherosclerosis inside of them as, through either lethargy or ignorance, they let their condition grow worse and worse without taking any of the steps to prolong their own lives.

A BIBLE CURE *Health Tip*
Dr. Colbert's Top Ten Cardiovascular Disease Risk Factors

1. Smoking
2. Elevated CRP levels
3. Elevated homocysteine levels

4. Elevated lipoprotein(a)
5. Elevated fibrinogen levels
6. Hypertension
7. Elevated cholesterol levels
8. Elevated triglycerides
9. Elevated blood sugar and insulin levels
10. Elevated lipoprotein phospholipase A2

Jesus said that we are to be in the world but not of it. (See John 17:11, 14–16.) Few realize that if we are to have the fullness of life God planned for us, this means the way we eat as well as our moral and kingdom-building conduct. At the moment, our standard American diet is killing us left and right. In order to counteract that, we need to learn to make wise dietary choices so that later we will still be living a healthy life when others may be either on the operating table, in a nursing home, or in the grave.

While the basic steps of eating a Mediterranean diet, regular exercise, taking proper supplements, and eliminating stress through living in God's peace and joy can address most of the risk factors of cardiovascular disease, there are certain adjustments you need to make to your regimen when particular risk factors affect your loved ones or you. The reason for this is that any one of these factors, while you take care of the rest, can still cause cardiovascular disease. For that reason alone, you need to be aware of them and ask your doctor about them the next time you have a checkup.

As I have studied cardiovascular disease over the years, I have found that there are no fewer than twenty-four individual risk factors that can lead to atherosclerotic heart disease. The list below begins with my top ten risk factors. They are the most dangerous. If I could print them in red ink for extra warning to you, I would! The last fourteen are in no particular order but are still life threatening. Each of them must specifically be addressed, or else you are just prolonging the countdown rather than defusing the bomb.

Also, please note that because of the importance of addressing cardiovascular disease in our nation, research continues every day revealing new breakthroughs and information that can be crucial in defeating heart disease for yourself or your loved ones. For that reason, please use the information here as a starting point and not necessarily a strict treatment regimen. Such specifics should be worked out between yourself and your doctor, as he or she should have the latest information available that bolsters your hope in preventing heart disease.

DR. COLBERT'S TOP TEN RISK FACTORS OF CARDIOVASCULAR DISEASE

1. Smoking

The most important lifestyle modification in preventing atherosclerosis is to get away from the air pollution of smoking. If you're a smoker, it's time to stop smoking! Secondly, whether you smoke or not, avoid secondhand smoke. Cigarette smoke fills the air with over four thousand different chemicals, fifty of which have been proven to be cancer causing. Further, these chemicals trigger significant free-radical reactions that may damage the lining of the arteries. They also damage healthy cholesterol and form oxidized cholesterol, which leads to more plaque formation. Smoking also causes blood platelets to clump together and also raises fibrinogen levels, which increases your risk of both heart attack and stroke.

The bottom line is that smoking sets you up for cardiovascular disease, cancer, and other degenerative diseases. It is imperative that you take steps today to get cigarettes and cigarette smoke out of your life for good—and that includes secondhand smoke.

2. Elevated CRP levels

C-reactive protein (CRP) is both a marker of inflammation and a promoter of inflammation. Elevated CRP blood levels create a constant environment prone to inflammation within your entire body. When CRP levels are high, every cell in your body is vulnerable to the damaging effects of inflammation. When this chronic inflammation occurs in the blood vessels, it usually causes the atherosclerosis, which is the first step toward having a heart attack and stroke.

There are now blood tests that determine CRP levels. As we will discuss in chapter 6, numerous recent studies have shown that CRP is likely a better predictor of heart attack and stroke risk than traditional cholesterol tests alone. Those with elevated CRP levels but acceptable cholesterol levels are more likely to have heart attacks or strokes than those with high cholesterol but low CRP. Also, those with high CRP levels are less likely to survive when a heart attack or stroke does occur. I think we will be seeing more in the media in the coming years about testing CRP levels as an important means of detecting chronic cardiovascular risk.

CRP is produced in many cells of the body in response to the presence of the cytokines that promote inflammation. C-reactive protein is mainly produced by fat cells, especially belly fat, and the liver in response to excess interleukin-6—a cytokine. CRP is released by abdominal fat and then is dumped directly into the liver. As a result, those who are overweight or obese, especially those who have abdominal fat, often have significantly higher levels of CRP in their bloodstreams than do lean people.

CRP RANGES FOR MEN AND WOMEN

Men CRP (mg/L)	Relative Risk For:	
	Future MI (heart attack)	Future Stroke
>2.11	2.9	1.9
1.15–2.10	2.6	1.9
0.56–1.14	1.7	1.7
<0.55	1.0	1.0

Women CRP (mg/L)	Relative Risk for Future MI or Stroke
>7.3	5.5
3.8–7.3	3.5
1.5–3.7	2.7
<1.5	1.0

To reduce CRP levels, you should follow a Mediterranean diet and avoid foods high in saturated fats and trans fats. You should also avoid fried foods and foods that are high glycemic— or raise the blood sugar rapidly. Sweets, white bread, white rice, and instant potatoes are prime examples of high-glycemic foods. Instead, you can choose to eat foods high in fiber, such as raw almonds, lentils, beans, peas, seeds, nuts, apples, berries, and so forth. Again, eating a Mediterranean diet is one of the simplest ways to lower CRP as well as many other risk factors.

A superantioxidant found in French maritime pine bark or made from combinations of grape seed, pine bark, and red wine extract has been shown to lower CRP levels. Studies have shown oligomeric proanthocyanidins (OPCs) can lower CRP by 50 percent.[1] Most studies have used doses of 120 to 300 mg daily. (See appendix.)

Another way to address CRP levels is by taking daily supplements that include (see appendix):

- Fish oil, pharmaceutical grade (1,000 mg, two to three times a day)
- Coenzyme Q_{10} (ubiquinol) (100–200 mg a day)
- Pine bark extract and grape seed extract, or OPCs (120–300 mg a day)
- Red yeast rice, or LipiControl (1,200 mg, twice a day with food; see appendix)
- Irvingia extract (150 mg, twice a day)

3. Elevated homocysteine levels

Homocysteine is a toxic, plaque-forming amino acid that is produced from the amino acid methionine. Without adequate B vitamins (B_6, B_{12}, and folic acid), homocysteine begins building up in the body and triggers plaque formation, oxidation of cholesterol, and potentially blood clots. Elevated homocysteine is an independent risk factor for cardiovascular disease as well as dementia and Alzheimer's disease, osteoporosis, macular degeneration, depression, headaches, birth defects, and certain forms of cancer.

I believe levels need to be reduced to 8–10 mmol/L or lower (the lower the better to see significant improvement). Because of this, I recommend seeking these levels through diet, supplements, and lifestyle changes. Once again, the Mediterranean diet can have a significant effect on this risk factor because it is lower in meat consumption.

For other means of lowering homocysteine to an acceptable level, I recommend taking the following every day:

- Folic acid (800–1,600 mcg a day)
- Vitamin B_6 (10–40 mg a day)
- Vitamin B_{12} (200–1,000 mcg a day)
- Trimethylglycine (1,000–2,000 mg a day)

For most people, taking the above B vitamins or a comprehensive multivitamin will be enough to counteract elevated homocysteine levels, but some have trouble converting folic acid to its active form. For those, adding the bioactive folic acid (5-methyltetrahydrofolate [5-MTHF], the active form of folic acid) will go further in reducing homocysteine levels. Researchers have found that giving 5-MTHF to subjects increased the plasma folate concentration 700 percent better than those who took folic acids alone.[2] Trials and tests suggest that a desirable dosage should be 800–1,000 mcg daily. Note as well that this should be added to the above intake of B vitamins and should not replace them.

Those who have a continued problem with excessive

homocysteine levels should ask their doctor about having a genomic test done to see if you genetically have a problem with methylenetetrahydrofolate reductase (MTHFR) enzyme production. SNPs (single nucleotide polymorphisms) are genetic side roads that are responsible for the differences between all of us. SNPs can make our genes perform below their optimal level and may lead to disease. One of MTHFR's main functions is converting folic acid to its active form so that it can be used by our bodies and help reduce homocysteine levels. Thus, when you have this genetic deficiency, you will have a surplus of homocysteine. Genomic tests can determine if you have a genetic "error" or mutation in this gene, which is the most commonly known inherited risk for high homocysteine levels. Although these mutations do impair the regulation of homocysteine, maintaining adequate folic acid levels (through supplements like FolaPro, the bioactive form of folic acid, 5-MTHF) in your system will correct high homocysteine levels. (See appendix.)

4. Elevated lipoprotein(a)

Lipoprotein(a), or Lp(a), is a protein that helps to repair damage in the arterial walls, but excessive levels of it are a direct cause of plaque formation and blood clots that cause heart attacks and strokes. Lp(a) also magnifies other coronary risk factors as it affects the size and number of LDL particles. As many as one in five who have heart disease will have elevated Lp(a) levels, which will usually lead them to have heart attacks as early as their forties or fifties. Lp(a) is more atherogenic than oxidized cholesterol.

Most experts concur that Lp(a) levels of lower than 30 mg/dL will significantly reduce the risk of heart disease, though the best way to reduce it is still debated. It appears niacin can be effective in lowering high Lp(a) levels, but the dosage usually needs to be higher (usually 2,000–4,000 mg a day). This can be problematic because of niacin's unpleasant side effects of flushing, burning, and itching. I suggest taking niacin after breakfast and dinner and with low-dose (80 mg) aspirin. Start with one niacin after breakfast and one after dinner, and after two weeks, increase the dose to two niacin after breakfast and two after dinner. Have your liver functions checked after one month of this regimen. Recheck the Lp(a) level in three months, and if it is still elevated, gradually raise your dose of niacin up to 4,000 mg a day using the same protocol. Recheck your liver functions in one month, and recheck your Lp(a) in three months. You should also discuss bioidentical hormone therapy with your doctor since testosterone in men and bioidentical estrogen in women can reduce Lp(a) levels by up to 25 percent. Avoid all trans fats if you have elevated Lp(a).

Other supplements to consider adding to your daily vitamin, mineral, and nutrient regimen to regulate Lp(a) are:

- L-carnitine (500 mg, two to three times a day)
- Pharmaceutical grade fish oil (1 g, two to three times a day)
- Niacin (see dosage above)

5. Elevated fibrinogen level

Blood clots lead to heart attacks and strokes—killing more than 600,000 Americans every year. Fibrinogen is a principal clotting protein crucial when we are injured, but levels that are too high will also increase the likelihood of a blood clot forming and rapidly developing. When you have elevated fibrinogen levels, the balance is tipped in the favor of unnecessary—and potentially deadly—blood clot formation. Fibrinogen can also lodge in artery walls to promote atherosclerosis.

A healthy fibrinogen level would be less than 300 mg/dL. A recent study has shown that for every 100 mg/dL increment above this, you will nearly double the likelihood of having coronary heart disease.[3] Another study showed that it may be the only independent predictor of dying from a heart attack, as it highly correlated with those who passed away within forty-two months of having one.[4]

Foods high in fat and refined starches are the first building block that raises fibrinogen levels. Inactivity is a second one. Too much estrogen as well as excess homocysteine (which interferes with the natural breakdown of fibrinogen) will also increase it. Oddly enough, being cold also encourages its production.

The Mediterranean diet is again a great place to start in keeping fibrinogen levels where they should be. Low dose (81 mg) aspirin taken with food will help prevent blood clots. Again, limit foods high in saturated fats, and avoid trans fats.

As far as supplements go, I also recommend the following daily (see appendix):

- Pharmaceutical grade fish oil (1,000 mg, three times a day)
- Nattokinase (4,000 units a day, which is two 50-mg capsules twice a day; do not take if you are on Coumadin or Plavix)

- Pine bark and/or grape seed extract, or OPCs (120–300 mg a day)

- Bromelain extract (500 mg, two times a day on an empty stomach); this is available at your local health food store

- Lumbrokinase (take 20 mg, three times a day, thirty minutes before meals; do not take this with nattokinase except under a doctor's supervision). I recommend that you be under the care of a physician when using this product.

6. Hypertension

Blood pressure is an important risk factor for heart disease. It is easy to keep an eye on your blood pressure with blood pressure stations everywhere from the doctor's office to pharmacies and local supermarkets. Blood pressure is presented as a ratio between two numbers, the systolic pressure (the force on your blood vessel walls as your heart beats) and the diastolic pressure (the force against those walls as the heart relaxes between beats to fill with blood). So, a blood pressure test will give you a reading such as 117/76 (read "117 over 76"). Research has found that for every 20/10 mmHg increment over 115/75 mmHg, your risk of a heart attack *doubles*. An amazing 50 million Americans suffer from hypertension or high blood pressure, and nearly a third of them *don't even know it*. Many of these people display no symptoms at all, and hypertension often goes undiagnosed and untreated for years.

You need to know what your blood pressure is and whether it is too high or not. Left untreated, high blood pressure will make you a major risk for either a heart attack or a stroke. Imagine it as leaving the hose on in your front yard all of the time with the nozzle on the end of it closed. This actually happened to my hose. For a few weeks the hose appeared normal, but eventually the pressure damaged the hose wall and destroyed the hose. So the next time you see a blood pressure machine, stop and check it. If desired, ambulatory blood pressure monitors are even available that will record your blood pressure readings every fifteen minutes for twenty-four hours so that you can have a picture of your daily fluctuations and averages. Regular blood pressure screening can help you receive an early diagnosis and treatment, which will greatly reduce the risks of further complications.

A **BIBLE CURE** *Health Fact*

Categories for Blood Pressure Levels in Adults

- *Normal blood pressure* is a systolic blood pressure below 120, and diastolic blood pressure lower than 80.
- *Pre-hypertension* is defined as systolic blood pressure between 120 and 139, and diastolic blood pressure between 80 and 89.
- *Hypertension stage I* is defined as systolic blood pressure between 140 and 159, and diastolic between 90 and 99.
- *Hypertension stage II* is defined as systolic blood pressure greater than 160, and diastolic greater than 100.

As with most conditions involving the health of your cardio-vascular system, lifestyle choices can play a significant role in prevention and control of hypertension. These include cutting out smoking and eliminating alcohol, limiting stress, taking up regular aerobic exercise, achieving and maintaining a healthy weight and losing body fat, and cutting down on caffeine. Eating habits that contribute to hypertension include consuming too much salt, sugar (such as foods with added high-fructose corn syrup), high-glycemic foods (such as white bread, white rice, etc.), and saturated fats, while not eating enough fiber and not taking in enough potassium, magnesium, and calcium. Some doctors have seen blood pressure drop between 20 and 40 mmHg when people cut out wheat, corn, and cornstarch from their diets, not to mention weight loss, especially losing belly fat.

Your top priority in changing your diet to defeat hypertension is to increase your potassium intake and decrease your salt intake, because a diet high in sodium and low in potassium is closely associated with hypertension. You want to limit your salt intake to less than 1,500 mg a day. (A teaspoon of salt is about 2,300 to 2,400 mg. Also, a medium baked potato has only about 5 mg of sodium; however, when this same potato is made into potato chips, it has about 1,560 mg of sodium.) This is a challenge, because the processed foods that most Americans take in have *twice as much sodium as potassium*, when we should be taking in *five times as much potassium as sodium*.

The only way to insure this balance is to increase your intake of fruits and vegetables, and not canned vegetables that are high in sodium.[5] These provide essential fatty acids, fiber, potassium, calcium, magnesium, and vitamin C. Eating fresh, natural foods rich in nutrients will help lower blood pressure.

And why not start using a juicer? You can juice carrots, apples, parsley, and celery once or twice a day. Drink at least half a cup a day of organic celery juice, since it has been discovered that celery can lower blood pressure, and add back a tablespoon of the pulp, which is fiber.

Other foods that may help lower blood pressure include:

- Garlic, especially aged garlic
- Sea vegetables
- Pomegranate juice
- Celery

Another good way to get your potassium is to use the brand No Salt (or any other similar variety of salt substitute) that contains 530 mg of potassium per ⅙ teaspoon. The DASH (Dietary Approaches to Stop Hypertension) diet is specifically designed to address the problems of too much salt intake. Research has shown that the DASH diet can lower systolic pressure by eleven points and diastolic by six. I consider the DASH diet a good place to start, but it should go further to the Mediterranean diet to be a lifestyle change that will address the widest number of health concerns.

Other valuable nutrients that will aid in blood pressure reduction are L-arginine and L-citrulline. You can get these in foods such as almonds, dark chocolate (in small amounts), walnuts, melons, garbanzo beans, peanuts, and salmon.

If you are facing high blood pressure, lose belly fat and follow my book *Dr. Colbert's "I Can Do This" Diet*. You can also look for the following in your daily supplements. (See appendix.)

- L-arginine, 2,000–3,000 mg
- L-citrulline, 200–1,000 mg

- Pomegranate juice or capsule, 1 capsule or 2 ounces of juice twice a day
- Garlic, 4 g of fresh garlic per day is equal to 18,000 mcg (18 mg) of alliin
- Seaweed extract, 1,200 mg, 1 to 2 capsules twice a day
- Pharmaceutical grade fish oil, 1 g two to three times a day
- Grape seed extract and/or pine bark extract (OPCs), 120–300 mg day
- Celery, four celery stalks daily or the equivalent in celery juice with 1–2 tablespoons of pulp added back to juice

(Note: if your blood pressure remains high, please see your physician and start a blood pressure medication.)

> For God has not given us a spirit of fear and timidity, but of power, love, and self-discipline.
> —2 TIMOTHY 1:7

7. Improper cholesterol levels

While we have already discussed many new factors that contribute to cardiovascular disease, we cannot neglect the old ones. Cholesterol is still a primary concern when addressing heart health, and the standard lipid panel tests of total, LDL, and HDL cholesterol levels are still very valid indicators of risks for cardiovascular disease. Believe it or not, despite the bad press we usually hear about cholesterol, it does provide several important life-sustaining functions between the liver and the body's cells, when it is kept in proper balance. It is only when cholesterol gets outside of optimal ranges that it begins to pose a threat.

Overall, you want LDL (low-density lipoprotein) to be low (think of the first "L" as indicating "low") and your HDL (high-density lipoprotein) to be high (think of that "H" as representing you want it "high"). The reason for this is that LDL cholesterol is the plaque-producing enemy and HDL is very beneficial in reversing plaque. HDL will actually "mine" bad cholesterol out of the walls of your arteries and dispose of it in the liver in a process called "reverse cholesterol transport"—a very desirable process.

Research is finding that the cholesterol levels thought acceptable in the past have changed. The optimum range for HDL is 60 mg/dL or higher, while the desired level of LDL is less than 100 mg/dL, and if an individual has other risk factors for cardiovascular disease or has cardiovascular disease, most doctors try to get the LDL to 70 mg/dL or lower. The American Heart Association considers total cholesterol of 200 to 240 mg/dL to be of concern, and 240 mg/dL or higher to more than double the risk of heart attack or stroke. In my opinion, if you have other risk factors for cardiovascular disease or if you have cardiovascular disease and your LDL is above 100 mg/dL and your HDL is below 50 mg/dL, you need to take immediate steps to correct these levels.

Your first step in reducing your LDL is best addressed in your diet. Probably the most important dietary advice to lower cholesterol is to eliminate sugar, fruit juice, and high-glycemic foods such as white bread, white rice, and instant potatoes and to follow the guidelines in *Dr. Colbert's "I Can Do This" Diet*. When you eat sugary foods and beverages or high-glycemic foods, they spike your blood sugar and raise your insulin levels. High insulin levels trigger your liver to produce more cholesterol. Also avoid fried foods and foods with trans fats, refined carbohydrates, and a lot of sugar, including fruit juices. Limit saturated fats, choose smaller portions of lean meats and nonfat dairy products, and peel the skin off chicken and turkey. Adopt the Mediterranean diet and look for snacks or foods that are high in fiber. (See the previous chapter again for more details on both of these.) Follow *Dr. Colbert's "I Can Do This" Diet* to help you achieve and maintain a healthy weight, and add aerobic exercise to raise your HDL levels.

I also recommend that you supplement your diet daily with (see appendix):

- Niacin (lowers LDL cholesterol and raises HDL, or the good cholesterol). To avoid flushing, start with 500 mg after breakfast and 500 mg after dinner with one baby aspirin. Do this for two weeks, then increase the dose to 1,000 mg after breakfast and 1,000 mg after dinner with one baby aspirin. Have your liver functions checked in one month with your primary care physician and your lipid panel checked in three months.

- Soluble fiber such as PGX fiber (two to four capsules with each meal)

- Plant sterols, or Cardio-Edge (two 400-mg capsules after each meal)

- Red yeast rice, or LipiControl (1,200 mg twice a day; take CoQ_{10} [ubiquinol] with red yeast rice)

Lastly, I often recommend hormone therapy for patients with elevated LDL because many people have high cholesterol as a result of low estrogen, progesterone, pregnenolone, DHEA, or testosterone levels in the blood. In addition, cholesterol is the precursor to testosterone and other sex hormones in the body. Therefore, when testosterone is low (in men), their bodies compensate by creating more cholesterol. If you have high LDL cholesterol, ask your doctor about blood tests that can measure your levels of testosterone and other hormones, and then discuss bioidentical hormone replacement to restore your hormone levels to optimal ranges as part of your plan to decrease your risk of cardiovascular disease. (Because of the limited space and scope of this book, there is a good deal of new information concerning cholesterol and its effects that I have not been able to address in these pages. If you want more information on the topic, please see my book *The Bible Cure for High Cholesterol*.)

Oxidized LDL

The prime focus of most drug research concerning cardiovascular disease has been about lowering cholesterol levels, and that is about all you will hear in their ads on television. However, thousands of studies are now showing how oxidized LDL is much more dangerous and promotes virtually every stage of atherosclerosis; therefore, in addition to lowering its level, it is just as important to keep your LDL cholesterol from becoming oxidized. LDL cholesterol can become oxidized by free radicals. Oxidized cholesterol is more prone to stick to arterial walls and form foam cells that eventually form plaque. Commercial tests are not yet available to measure oxidized cholesterol at affordable prices. Since there is no economical test to determine the degree to which LDL cholesterol is oxidizing in your body, it is best to quench inflammation, take antioxidants, lower Apo B (apolipoprotein B) levels, and take supplements to reduce small LDL particles. Thankfully much of what I have already prescribed for you dietarily with antioxidants and exercise already address oxidation.

For example, the higher the calorie, sugar, and fat content of each of your meals, the greater you will experience what doctors call *postprandial oxidative stress* after you have finished eating. It is an oxidation process. So eating a Mediterranean diet wins again. You can also drink water with lemon or lime, green or black tea, or 2 ounces pomegranate juice with your meals to reduce this oxidation process.

I also suggest you take the following in supplement form if you are not getting these nutrients to lower oxidized cholesterol (see appendix):

- Gamma tocopherol (200–250 mg, once or twice a day with food)
- Pomegranate juice (2 ounces, twice a day)
- Ubiquinol (CoQ$_{10}$; 100–200 mg a day)
- Grape seed and/or pine bark extracts (120–300 mg, once or twice a day)
- Theaflavin (350 mg, once or twice a day)

Apolipoprotein B

Apo B is a measurement of the number of LDL (bad cholesterol) particles in the blood. It is the protein portion of the low-density lipoprotein and transfers cholesterol from the lipoprotein either to the cells to be used or to the liver to be excreted. If the amount of Apo B present is in proportion to the amount needed by the cells, then no problem occurs. However, if you have an excess of Apo B, the excess Apo B will usually deposit cholesterol in arterial walls. Apo B determines whether the cholesterol is used correctly, it determines if cholesterol is excreted in the liver, and it determines if cholesterol ends up as plaque. It is believed that LDL particle numbers may predict coronary artery disease risk better than LDL levels. Apo B is mainly genetically determined. Having a large number of LDL particles has been shown to increase heart attack risk even when the total LDL is normal or low and that this measurement is among the most powerful tools for predicting an ischemic event.

To determine the number of LDL particles, it is possible to count apolipoprotein B (Apo B) particles, because Apo B is the major protein particle of an LDL cluster, and each LDL cluster will have only one. It is possible to have an LDL number of 80 (normal), for instance, but an Apo B count of either 50 (normal) or 130 (elevated). (Note that a normal Apo B level would be anything below 60.) Unfortunately, a low LDL amount but a high Apo B count is fairly common and increases your risk of cardiovascular disease.

Proper diet, regular exercise, and supplementation are effective in reducing your Apo B level. Avoiding trans fats and reducing saturated fats in your diet are also extremely important in lowering Apo B. Below are supplements to lower Apo B (see appendix):

- Niacin (2–4 g a day; see instructions on page 35)
- Red yeast rice (1,200 mg, twice a day)
- Sytrinol (in Cardio-Edge; two with each meal)
- Pantethine (900–1,200 mg a day)

LDL particle size:

Small LDL particles are far more atherogenic (plaque forming) because they are 40 percent more likely to get stuck in artery walls and form plaque. Studies have shown small LDL triples the likelihood of developing coronary plaque. Small LDL also shows a tendency toward insulin resistance and thus an increased risk of diabetes, especially if you are overweight or obese. Other research has shown that if you have small LDL particles and high C-reactive protein (CRP) levels, your chances of a heart attack are six times higher than normal.

The best way to keep LDL particle size larger and safer is by maintaining a healthy weight. Refer to my book *Dr. Colbert's "I Can Do This" Diet*. Taking 1,500–3,000 mg of niacin a day (or as directed by your doctor) can also help control LDL size. Research is showing niacin may be the most effective nutrient to take to help eliminate small LDL. It is also best to eat foods that have a low glycemic index (GI) number and thus release sugars more slowly after eating. Note that statin drugs have only a minimal to no effect on LDL particle size. Taking soluble fiber supplements such as PGX fiber with your other foods can also help in promoting larger LDL particles, as can making sure you are getting enough omega-3 fatty acids and getting regular exercise.

Here are some supplements to improve LDL particle size (see appendix):

- Niacin (1,500–3,000 mg a day; see instructions on page 35)
- Pharmaceutical grade fish oil (two to three times a day)
- Soluble fiber such as PGX fiber (two to four capsules with each meal, taken with 8–16 ounces of water or other beverage)

Low HDL cholesterol

High-density lipoprotein (HDL) helps perform many beneficial functions that protect against atherosclerosis. At its best, HDL will help reverse atherosclerosis by taking cholesterol out of the walls of your arteries and out of plaque and disposing of it in the liver in a process known as reverse cholesterol transport. Recent research has also found that the larger these molecules are, the more effective they are in this process.

HDL particle size: Just as larger LDL particles are healthier for you, so are larger HDL particles, because larger HDL is better at the "reverse cholesterol transport," which actually takes the cholesterol out of plaque in artery walls. HDL2 is the most efficient HDL particle for reverse cholesterol transport. While this test will specifically tell you the size of your HDL particles if that is a concern to you, the good news is that the higher your HDL cholesterol is in standard cholesterol tests, the more likely it is that you also have large HDL particles.

While healthy weight is again crucial, strictly low-fat diets will reduce your HDL and its particles' size. This is why the Mediterranean diet, which includes fats in monounsaturated form, is better than calorie-reduction diets. Strategies that increase LDL particle size will also increase HDL particle size.

For HDL to perform its most vital functions, it must have an enzyme called paraoxonase 1 (PON 1) attached to it. However, as we get older, PON 1 decreases. Thus even if your HDL levels are great, your HDL will not be as effective as it could be without also raising your PON 1. PON 1 is crucial not just to vascular health but also to preventing diabetes, strokes, arthritis, and certain forms of cancer because it works as both an antioxidant and an anti-inflammatory agent. Low serum PON 1 levels can even be an independent risk factor for heart disease. The good news is that you don't need an expensive drug to encourage your liver to produce more PON 1. The most recent studies show that pomegranate and its extracts significantly boost both PON 1 levels and PON 1 activity.

In a recent study in Israel, researchers found that after only two weeks of consuming pomegranate juice daily, test subjects had a 20 percent increase in PON 1 activity and a markedly reduced amount of the LDL "clumping" that leads to the formation of foam cells. Pomegranate juice and its extracts boosted the outflow of cholesterol by 39 percent. After a year in the study, subjects realized an 83 percent increase in PON 1 and a 90 percent decrease in oxidized LDL. While the artery flow of the placebo group narrowed by 9 percent, the test group saw a 30 percent reversal of narrowing in the arteries.[6] Because of this evidence, I highly recommend adding 400–500 mg of standardized pomegranate extract or its equivalent, 2–4 ounces of pomegranate juice twice a day, to your daily diet.

Since excess abdominal fat appears to contribute to low HDL, I suggest not only reaching and staying at your healthy weight but also adding regular physical activity and aerobic exercise to encourage higher HDL levels. So make room in your schedule for regular aerobic exercise.

I also suggest daily supplementing your diet with the following (see appendix):

- Niacin (1,000 mg, two times a day after breakfast and dinner with one baby aspirin; see protocol on page 35 to avoid the niacin flush)
- Quercetin (200–400 mg, three times daily)
- Resveratrol (175–500 mg a day)
- Pomegranate (400 mg, two times a day, or 2–4 ounces, two times a day, of pomegranate juice)

Bioidentical hormone therapy is also something you should consider if your HDL levels are not improved. I also may add more niacin, up to 2,000 mg, after breakfast, and 2,000 mg after dinner. Gradually increase the dose and take one or more enteric-coated aspirins with the niacin to avoid the flushing. I also check liver function tests each month while increasing the dose of niacin.

8. Elevated triglycerides

Triglycerides are the chemical form of most fats as they exist within the body. Calories that are not immediately burned may also be converted into triglycerides and stored in the fat deposits throughout our bodies, especially in abdominal fat. Like excess cholesterol, excess triglycerides will contribute to the buildup of plaque in the walls of our arteries, thus increasing the risk of atherosclerosis. Continually high triglyceride levels can also cause other unwanted complications. For example, it predisposes individuals to type 2 diabetes and its related complications as well as dementia and a legion of dangerous inflammatory diseases.

In the decades past it was believed that triglyceride levels below 149 mg/dL were safe, but more recent studies are suggesting the fasting (taken twelve or more hours after last eating) level of triglycerides should be below 100 mg/dL, and optimally below 80 mg/dL for healthy individuals. If you have a history of cardiovascular disease, then an even lower 60 mg/dL or less should be your goal. Non-fasting levels (taken two to eight hours after eating) should be under 116 mg/dL. The higher these levels, the higher the risk of having a cardiovascular event.

Again, the best place to start in addressing this risk is to modify what you eat. Avoid sugars and high-glycemic foods that raise the blood sugar quickly. Those foods and beverages also raise the triglyceride levels. Instead, choose foods that are on the Mediterranean diet, but for more specific information, the University of Sydney manages a Web site about the glycemic index of foods at www.glycemicindex.com. The glycemic index (GI) gives an indicator of the rate at which different carbohydrates and foods break down to release sugar into the bloodstream. Glucose has a GI of 100, and most refined carbohydrates such as white bread, white rice, and instant potatoes, have a high GI. The range of the glycemic index is 0 to 100. Even juices and smoothies that seem to be healthy can raise your triglyceride levels as well as your blood sugar. The glycemic index applies only to carbohydrates and sugars and not proteins and fats. Processed foods and those high in carbohydrates have higher GIs and tend to elevate the triglycerides. According to the University of Sydney site just mentioned, foods that have a GI of 70 or higher are considered high, and 55 or lower are considered low-glycemic foods. In fact, foods with little or no carbohydrates in them will have a GI of 0 to 1, such as broccoli.

Ingesting soluble fiber, such as PGX, before, during, or after your meals or eating foods high in fiber will lower the glycemic index of those foods, as it delays the absorption of carbohydrates and sugars and prevents the rapid rise in blood sugar. Also avoid deep-fried foods such as french fries, chips, fried chicken, fried fish, and doughnuts, and avoid all trans fats, as these will raise triglyceride levels. Decrease intake of polyunsaturated fats such as most salad dressings, cream-based soups, gravies, and sauces. Restrict or avoid alcohol since this also raises triglyceride levels.

Fish oil or omega-3 capsules are also an effective way to reduce triglycerides. A good dosage for most people would be 1,000 mg, three times a day, but if your triglyceride levels are high, I would increase the dose to 4,000 or 5,000 mg in divided doses. If you are taking the higher amount, have your blood retested every two or three months to ensure your dosage is having the proper effect.

Niacin (2,000 to 3,000 mg every day, usually in divided doses after breakfast and dinner to avoid flushing) can also significantly lower triglycerides, as well as address high total and LDL cholesterol and low HDL. Niacin can have an unpleasant skin flushing, burning, and itching side effect, so again I suggest taking it after meals two times a day and with low-dose (80 mg) aspirin (one to three with each dose) to avoid or minimize flushing.

9. Elevated blood sugar and elevated insulin level

As we age, gain weight, and continue poor eating habits, our cells and tissues become less sensitive to the effects of insulin in our body, and this causes our blood sugar to gradually rise rather than the sugar being effectively absorbed into our cells to be burned as fuel. The main cause of this is obesity, lack of exercise, poor diet, and the sharp decline in hormones that we experience as we get older, which are critical for insulin sensitivity. The more belly fat, typically the more insulin resistance, and this usually eventually leads to prediabetes or diabetes.

While it was once thought fasting blood glucose levels up to 125 mg/dL were acceptable, more recent studies suggest that anything over 85 mg/dL will incrementally add to your risk of a cardiovascular event. Even lower than that—75 mg/dL or less—is more likely to be an ideal fasting glucose number. What is nice is that addressing fasting glucose will also affect fasting insulin levels, LDL, total cholesterol, triglycerides, and CRP levels.

Again, the best place to start is with a healthy diet and regular exercise to keep your metabolism functioning at an optimal level. I especially recommend losing belly fat by following my program in *Dr. Colbert's "I Can Do This" Diet*. Taking soluble dietary fiber (such as PGX fiber, two to four capsules before each meal) will also help lower your blood sugar and cholesterol levels. For more information, see *The New Bible Cure for Diabetes*. Including the following with your daily supplements will also help control insulin and glucose levels:

- Chromium picolinate (400 mcg, twice a day, or up to 1,000 mcg a day)

- PGX soluble fiber (2–4 capsules with 8–16 ounces of water before each meal)
- Cinnamon extract, such as Cinnulin (175 mg before each meal)
- Vitamin D (2,000–6,000 IU a day depending on your blood level of vitamin D_3)
- Alpha lipoic acid (300 mg, twice a day)
- Omega-3 fatty acids (EPA/DHA; 1,000 mg, two to three times a day)
- Testosterone in men if their blood levels are low and bioidentical transdermal estrogen and progesterone cream in women in a balanced ratio if levels are low
- Irvingia extract (150 mg, or two capsules, twice a day)

10. Elevated lipoprotein phospholipase A2

Lipoprotein phospholipase A2 (Lp-PLA2) is the enzyme that is found in high concentration in plaque that is ready to rupture or unstable plaque and is associated with inflammation in the plaque. Elevated levels of Lp-PLA2 may well signal that atherosclerotic plaque is growing more susceptible to rupturing and thus raises the chance of a sudden blood clot that could lead to a heart attack or stroke.

It is an indicator of inflammation that directly promotes rupture-prone plaque, and thus is also evidence that a dangerous blood clot is likely to occur. In the autopsies of twenty-five patients who had died from sudden coronary events, areas with early plaque formations showed little Lp-PLA2, while the ruptured plaque areas that had caused death showed intense levels of Lp-PLA2.[7]

Because of this, testing for Lp-PLA2 concentration can be a key indicator of how likely you are to experience a sudden cardiovascular event. Lp-PLA2 levels rise in people at risk for a stroke or heart attack. This testing can be done with a simple blood test called a PLAC test, which is easy and inexpensive and may save your life. It is also less affected by viral and other infections than are C-reactive protein tests. As such, it is also a good tool to monitor the effects of changing your diet, of your daily supplements, and of how your cardiovascular health changes as you exercise more, stop smoking, or address the other risk factors we have explored in this chapter. The normal level is a Lp-PLA2 less than 200, and greater than 235 is indicative of greater risk of heart attack or stroke. Those with high Lp-PLA2 are twice as likely to suffer a heart attack and five times as likely to suffer a stroke. When CRP and Lp-PLA2 are both elevated, the numbers are doubled again. Follow the recommend diet and supplements for lowering CRP to lower Lp-PLA2 levels.

OTHER RISK FACTORS OF CARDIOVASCULAR DISEASE

11. Alcohol

Drinking alcoholic beverages can raise triglycerides—a harmful type of fat—in your bloodstream as well as increase calorie intake and risk of high blood pressure. While not drinking at all is preferred by many, there are some positive effects that can be derived from drinking a glass of red wine with dinner. Red wine has been shown to contain flavonoids and other antioxidants, including resveratrol, that help raise HDL cholesterol, prevent blood clots, and help prevent cardiovascular disease. However, according to the American Heart Association, "No direct comparison trials have been done to determine the specific effect of wine or other alcohol on the risk of developing heart disease or stroke."[8]

So, if you do choose to drink alcohol, do so only in moderation, which means two drinks or fewer for men and one or fewer for women. (A drink is one 12-ounce beer, 4 ounces of wine, 1.5 ounce of 80-proof spirits, or 1 ounce of 100-proof spirits.) I also suggest drinking only with meals and, if you do drink, to choose red wine. Personally, I do not recommend drinking any alcohol at all since too many people find it difficult to stop after only one or two glasses. However, one capsule of Living Resveratrol has the health benefits of 600 glasses of red wine. So, if you choose not to drink, as I do, Living Resveratrol will give you all the benefits of red wine without the drawbacks.

12. Low testosterone levels in men and low estrogen levels in women

As we grow older, both men and women produce fewer sex hormones (for men, that's less testosterone, and for women, especially after menopause, less estrogen and progesterone). One crucial problem of low sex hormone production is it is associated with inflammation. Thus it increases the risk of atherosclerosis and susceptibility to blood clots. Men have additional risks because abdominal fat will produce excess aromatase, which will turn testosterone into estrogen, and excess estrogen in aging men has been tied to higher levels of C-reactive protein in the blood, thus greater inflammation, causing more plaque. Testosterone is also a crucial player in the reverse cholesterol transport process. As one study stated, "In men selected for coronary arteriography, age, HDL, and free testosterone may be stronger predictors of degree of coronary artery disease than are blood pressure, cholesterol, diabetes, smoking, and body mass index (BMI)."[9]

Hormone therapy is also potentially risky, as giving oral estrogen to women after menopause can actually increase the risk of heart disease, whereas transdermal dosing helps prevent cardiovascular disease. Bioidentical hormone replacement therapy should be done under the supervision of a physician trained in bioidentical hormone replacement therapy. (See appendix.)

Men can counteract excess aromatase in their systems by taking plant lignans such as ground flaxseeds (2 tablespoons, one to two times a day) and having their compounding pharmacist add chrysin to the testosterone cream. In the long run, losing belly fat is an important part of keeping testosterone levels higher and estrogen lower in men. Restrict or avoid alcohol consumption since it will inhibit the liver's ability to remove excess estrogen.

13. Low vitamin D_3 levels

Within the last decade, in addition to its protective attributes for bones, vitamin D_3 has also been recognized as a key protector against heart disease. A study from 2004 showed that men with low vitamin D_3 levels were twice as likely as men with normal levels to suffer heart attacks.[10] Vitamin D_3 aids vascular health in many different ways, one of the most important of which is its reduction of the chronic inflammatory reactions associated with atherosclerosis.

Getting enough vitamin D_3 is also one of the easiest deficiencies to address, since our bodies can usually produce it on their own if we get the minimum sunlight every day. However, as we age, we lose the ability to adequately convert sunlight to vitamin D_3, and too much sunlight may predispose us to skin cancers, including melanoma, basal cell carcinoma, and squamous cell carcinoma. It is not so with vitamin D_3 supplements, however. I recommend either taking 2,000–6,000 IU of vitamin D_3 every day, depending on your vitamin D_3 lab test, or getting the equivalent in sunshine, which would be about fifteen to twenty minutes of sunshine a day if cleared by your doctor. A vitamin D_3 level below 32 ng/ml is considered low; however, I try to get my patients vitamin D_3 level in the optimal range, which is 50–100 ng/ml.

14. Low vitamin K_2 levels

The "K" in vitamin K_2 is derived from the German word *koagulation*, because of the vitamin's importance in blood clotting in case of an injury. However, a secondary benefit of vitamin K_2 is that it regulates proteins in the bloodstream that guide calcium to deposit into the bones rather than in artery walls. Thus it is an important compound for preventing arterial calcification, chronic inflammation, and in lowering the risk of heart attacks.

Being deficient in vitamin K_1 is not common for a number of reasons. One reason is that it is widespread in ordinary foods such as green, leafy vegetables. Vitamin K_2 is present in egg yolks, dairy products, and organ meats, all of which raise cholesterol levels and is therefore commonly deficient in many Americans at risk for heart disease. In areas of Japan, a dish called natto, which is fermented soybeans, is usually eaten a few times a week. It is high in vitamin K_2 and especially the MK-7 type of vitamin K_2. According to the 2004 Rotterdam Heart Study that followed 4,800 subjects for seven years, the subjects that ate the most vitamin K_2 in their diet had a 57 percent reduction in death from cardiovascular disease. This study suggested that vitamin K_2 gives cardiovascular benefits by inhibiting arterial calcification.[11]

Those most at risk for vitamin K deficiency are those taking anticoagulant drugs (such as Coumadin), who are unable to take vitamin K or foods containing vitamin K, or individuals who have liver damage or disease.[12] Research has also shown that people who have fat malabsorption disorders may also be at risk of low vitamin K levels.[13] I recommend 1,000 mcg a day of vitamin K_2 unless you are taking Coumadin. Consult with your physician.

15. Low nitric oxide

Since there are really no economical tests to determine nitric oxide levels in our bloodstream, as we age we should all do what we can to address our bodies' decreasing ability to produce the nitric oxide our blood vessels need to remain pliable and healthy. Proper levels of nitric oxide protect the structural integrity of the endothelium (the innermost layer of a blood vessel or artery) and keep blood vessels contracting and dilating with youthful flexibility. Since the two prime causes of heart attack and stroke are the occlusion of an artery from a blood clot due to atherosclerosis combined with endothelial dysfunction *and* abnormal platelet activation, maintaining nitric oxide levels in a healthy range is a key component of slowing or preventing these activities. Nitric oxide slows the accumulation of plaque, helps prevent blood clots, and even helps to lower the blood pressure.

Nitric oxide also helps maintain proper blood pressure because blood vessel contraction and expansion help regulate this flow. (Think of this functioning like a garden hose with a nozzle on one end—if you need to get higher pressures, you decrease the circumference of the hole on the nozzle; if you need lower pressure, you increase the circumference of the nozzle—"youthful" blood vessels expand and contract similar to this.)

A BIBLE CURE Health Fact

Erectile dysfunction due to low nitric oxide levels is usually a signal of cardiovascular disease. Patients usually experience erectile dysfunction four or five years prior to developing symptoms of cardiovascular disease.

Raw almonds, peanuts, walnuts, garbanzo beans, dark chocolate, salmon, and lean red meat are all known to enhance the production of nitric oxide in our bodies. Foods containing polyphenols—fruits mainly—also protect against oxidation. You can receive polyphenols through drinking cocoa, tea, or a small amount of pomegranate juice or red wine with your meals. I also encourage eating antioxidant foods such as blueberries, blackberries, raspberries, and red grapes, as we have already described in the Mediterranean diet. Exercise elevates levels of the enzyme nitric oxide synthase that produces nitric oxide in the body and promotes continuous production of nitric oxide by the endothelial cells.

I also suggest paying attention to foods that are rich in L-arginine and L-citrulline, which help blood flow and improve the healthy functioning of endothelial cells. Examples of these include raw almonds, dark chocolate (in small amounts), walnuts, melons, garbanzo beans, peanuts, and salmon. I personally take a handful of raw almonds twice a day. If you desire supplements to boost nitric oxide, I recommend L-arginine (4–6 g at bedtime) and L-citrulline (200–600 mg at bedtime) or ProArgi-9 from Synergy. (See appendix.)

16. Low blood EPA/DHA

It is no news that scientists have documented markedly lower rates of heart attacks among populations that eat a lot of cold-water fish such as salmon, mackerel, lake trout, herring, sardines, and tuna. The reason for this is that these fish are high in omega-3 acids, specifically the EPA and DHA forms. Studies have found that independent of any other risk factors, low EPA/DHA levels increase the risk of a heart attack, suffering from angina, or experiencing a stroke. Compared to other age-equivalent groups, research has shown that the risk of unstable angina and heart attack are reduced 62 percent for every 1.24 percent increase of whole-blood EPA/DHA.[14]

Two or more meals a week including cold-water fish can make a marked decrease in the risk of a heart attack. However, I also suggest that regular pharmaceutical grade omega-3 capsules at least 1,000 mg, two times a day, be included in your daily supplement routine. A higher dosage may be warranted if you have certain other issues such as high triglycerides.

One word of caution: not all nutritional supplements are created equal. In that same way that people will strip-mine the countryside for a metal or cut corners manufacturing a product, people will cut corners in producing supplements that are of high enough quality to give you the proper benefits. Fish oil capsules are among the worst violators of quality control. I recommend a pharmaceutical grade fish oil that is free of mercury and other contaminates. Also, taste it to make sure it's not rancid. Rancid fish oil will create more oxidative stress and predispose you to heart disease. We now have a blood test that can measure the level of EPA and DHA in the blood.

17. Heavy metal toxicity

In our modern, industrial world, toxic heavy metals have seeped into our water, food, air, and cookware, not to mention our workplaces. While cold-water fish are great sources of omega-3 fatty acids, they are also often sources of toxic mercury that slowly builds up in our bodies. "Silver" or amalgam dental fillings are generally 49–53 percent mercury, and I have had patients develop troubling symptoms because they were absorbing too much mercury from such fillings. We extract over a billion tons of lead each year. Lead content in the bones of healthy people is one hundred times greater than one hundred years ago. Lead, aluminum, arsenic, cadmium, beryllium, copper, iron, and nickel are so prevalent they are impossible to avoid, and a buildup of them causes a host of physical problems, not the least of which is cardiovascular disease. Especially lead, cadmium, and mercury are the most toxic to our cardiovascular health. These toxic metals cause free radicals and oxidative stress, deactivate valuable minerals, and poison different protective enzyme systems.

Your first step is to do what you can to limit your toxin intake. Eat living, organic foods, free-range lean meats, and low-fat organic dairy products. Filter your water or find clean, pure spring sources. Avoid air pollution and secondhand smoke—walk along trails or in parks instead of along streets or roadways. Wear rubber gloves when cleaning, and look for natural cleaning alternatives and natural personal care products.

The only real answer to this problem beyond that is regular detoxification. One method is chelation therapy (see chapter 4), which uses a substance called ethylenediaminetetraacetic acid (EDTA) to remove these heavy metals from your body. (EDTA should only be used under the supervision of a physician.) While the AHA does not endorse it as a treatment for cardiovascular disease, chelation therapy does help remove toxic metals, which will improve endothelial cell health and increase the amount of nitric oxide produced. These toxic heavy metals may also create excessive oxidation of LDL cholesterol, one of the main causes of atherosclerosis. Mercury deactivates selenium, which is important for glutathione regeneration. Glutathione is our bodies' most important antioxidant, and mercury inhibits glutathione. Glutathione reduces inflammation and helps prevent cardiovascular disease. (See appendix.) There will be more about chelation therapy in the next chapter.

Zeolites are simply microporous inorganic minerals formed from volcanic ash and sea salt over millions of years. The microporous honeycomb-type structures contain channels or openings where heavy metals and minerals can bind. The aluminum building block carries a negative charge that attracts positive minerals, including calcium, magnesium, potassium, and sodium. These positive minerals can then be displaced by heavy metals such as mercury, lead, cadmium, and so forth. (See appendix.)

The herb cilantro has also been shown to have some wonderful chelation properties and is available in supplement form. Cilantro chelates mercury, lead, aluminum, asbestos, and cadmium. (For more information on this topic, refer to my books *What You Don't Know May Be Killing You*, *The Seven Pillars of Health*, and *Toxic Relief*.)

18. Excessive stress

Are you a type A personality? You are if you're often impatient, extremely competitive, and consistently aggressive in most everything you do. Research shows that type A individuals with high hostility have twice the risk of heart disease than non–type A folks. We know that constant excessive anger, worry, stress, and anxiety raise adrenaline levels, raise blood pressure, and thereby stress the heart and circulatory system. The risk of heart disease—especially heart attack—increases for the type A types. Isn't it interesting that the majority of heart attacks occur on Monday morning, when many are dreading work?

Comedian Lily Tomlin put it nicely: "The trouble with the rat race is that even if you win, you're still a rat." Many of us are so caught up in the race to get ahead that we leave our health behind. Our hearts suffer under the stress and tension of trying to be on top and at the head of every line.

Type A personalities are always in a hurry, trying to accomplish too many activities or check off too many tasks in too little an amount of time. They tend to accelerate daily activities (speeding up speech and finishing the sentences of others in a conversation, walking and eating quickly, doing two or three tasks at the same time) and often engage in two or more conversations all at once. Unfortunately, they also develop a drive that is self-destructive (usually unconsciously).[15] They look forward to someday escaping life's treadmill and retiring early, but too many of them never make it as they tend to spend their health to make money, and then spend their retirement using their money to try to get back their health. The most destructive characteristic of type A behavior is hostility. Hostility includes anger and bitterness, which are very damaging to one's blood vessels.

The best ways to cope with stress are practicing gratitude, getting ten belly laughs a day, incorporating margin in your life, practicing forgiveness every day, and walking in love toward everyone, no matter how they treat you. For more information on this topic, refer to *Deadly Emotions*, *Stress Less*, and *The Seven Pillars of Health*.

Studies have supported what has long been known from Proverbs 17:22: "A cheerful heart is good medicine, but a broken spirit saps a person's strength." Laughter has amazing healing qualities, as does caring for others. Even owning a pet has been shown to have positive health benefits. Don't rush through life trying to get to the end only to find you didn't really live along the way. Jesus promised us a full, abundant life, and He never intended that it would only be after you retired!

19. Deadly emotions, including depression

It should not be surprising to you that the "heartsickness" of clinical depression—and chronically experiencing negative emotions such as anger, resentment, unforgiveness, and hostility—will actually have repercussions for your physical heart. Depressed people suffer four times the risk of heart disease that nondepressed people do. Cardiovascular disease and depression actually share biochemical similarities. The flip side of this is that sometimes the two can be addressed together through what we eat and the supplements we take.

Those who experience chronic hopelessness and sadness tend to have more inflammatory proteins in their systems such as C-reactive protein and interleukin-1 beta. Depression also increases the release of stress hormones that over time will contribute to hypertension, insulin resistance, and diabetes. They also tend to have higher levels of homocysteine, increased oxidative stress, and lower levels of omega-3 fatty acids and folic acid (so look to add these to your supplements in the dosages recommended elsewhere in this chapter).

A **BIBLE CURE** Health Fact

Anxiety is also associated with cardiovascular disease. Research shows that men with high anxiety levels are up to six times more likely to experience sudden cardiac death than nonanxious men.

Though it is not known exactly why, depressed people tend to exercise less, smoke more, eat less nutritiously, and not follow their prescriptions as well. Thus they also seem to have more problems with weight control. (For more information on depression and anxiety, please refer to my book *The New Bible Cure for Depression and Anxiety*.)

20. Excess belly fat

As we have already discussed in several of these sections, maintaining your ideal body weight is one of the most important factors in addressing a majority of the risk factors included in this chapter. Belly fat is particularly troublesome because it produces excessive amounts of inflammatory compounds, such as CRP, that increase your risk of cardiovascular disease. If you need to lose weight, I recommend you pick up a copy of my book *Dr. Colbert's "I Can Do This" Diet*.

A **BIBLE CURE** *Health Tip*
Keys for Weight Loss

- Remove all irresistible foods from the house, including cookies, chips, and ice cream.

- Drink two quarts of filtered or bottled water every day. It is best to drink two 8-ounce glasses thirty minutes before each meal, or one to two 8-ounce glasses two and a half hours after each meal. It's especially important to drink 8–16 ounces glasses of water upon awakening.

- Consult your doctor about getting on a regular exercise program.

- Avoid sugar.

- You may eat fruit; however, avoid fruit juices and smoothies.

- Avoid alcohol, but if you must drink, drink only one to two 4-ounce glasses of red wine if you are male, and only one 4-ounce glass if you are female.

- Avoid all fried foods and trans fats.

- Dramatically decrease or avoid high-glycemic starches, especially for the evening meal. Starches include all breads; crackers; bagels; potatoes; pasta; rice; corn; and black, pinto, and red beans. Also limit intake of bananas.

- Eat fresh fruits; steamed, stir-fried, or raw vegetables; lean, free-range meats; and salads.

- Fiber supplements, such as PGX fiber (two to four capsules), before each meal will help decrease your appetite and stabilize your blood sugar.

- Do not eat dinner past 7:00 p.m.
- Before meals, eat large, colorful salads without croutons and with minimal cheese and a salad spritzer.
- Eat broth-based vegetable soup (low in sodium) before meals.
- Eat a well-balanced diet with 40 percent high-fiber carbs, 30 percent free-range lean protein, and 30 percent healthy fats. (See my book *Dr. Colbert's "I Can Do This" Diet*.)

21. Genetic factors

As has long been known, risk of cardiovascular disease can be passed down from generation to generation. If your parents and grandparents suffered from cardiovascular disease, it is all the more important that you take significant steps to counteract it throughout your lifetime, especially once you reach your forties and fifties. Proper diet, exercise, and supplements should already be part of your daily routine.

However, researchers are finding out more and more about what it is exactly in our genetic makeup that predisposes us to heart disease and risk of strokes. Two main candidates at this writing are the apolipoprotein E gene (APOE) and the KIF family of genes that are important to making the kinesin proteins that transport other proteins within a variety of bodily systems.

The APOE gene comes in three variations: APOE3 is considered the "normal" variation of the gene and appears in about 64 percent of the population; APOE2 and APOE4 are considered dysfunctional forms of the gene, and both of these are linked to atherosclerosis. APOE4 is found in around 25 percent of the population and is also linked to Alzheimer's disease and impaired cognitive function. APOE2 is linked to hyperlipidemia (which is more rare and only happens in about 11 percent of Americans), a condition that tends toward higher levels of cholesterol and the other lipids that inspire atherosclerosis.

Such predispositions are not a death sentence; however, the treatment suggestions you have already read earlier in this chapter can address these. It just becomes more important to do so if you have one of these genetic conditions. People with the APOE4 gene need to be on a very low-fat diet, or 20 percent of their total calories. They should avoid trans fats and fried foods and restrict saturated and polyunsaturated fats. The fats they should choose should be mainly monounsaturated fates, such as olive oil, almonds, avocados, and omega-3 fats such as fatty fish and flaxseeds. People with APOE4 typically have an elevated cholesterol level and are at an increased risk of cardiovascular disease and Alzheimer's disease. (Also see chapter 6 for more information on genomic testing for APOE variants and what to do about them.)

One of the KIF family gene variations, the kinesin-like protein 6 (KIF6), has been shown in three recent majors studies to have adverse effects on cardiovascular risk. More research needs to be done in these areas about how these genes actually raise this risk, but such research also shows great promise for better understanding the formation of atherosclerosis and better ways to treat the diseases in the future. If you test positive for this gene variant (again, see chapter 6 for more on this testing), most doctors put patients on statin drugs. I always recommend adding ubiquinol (living CoQ_{10}, 100 mg a day) since statins may deplete the body of CoQ_{10}.

Other genomic tests to see if you are at risk of having a blood clot is the genomic test for Factor II and Factor V.

While genomic testing is available to see if you have these

tendencies, it is still important just to know your family history and its tendencies toward heart disease. Do what you can in the meantime as more research in these areas come up with more specific treatments. Until then, I suggest following the suggestions throughout this chapter for lowering your cholesterol as well as defeating the other risk factors that will all have benefits for fighting these genetic predispositions as well. (See the screening tests in chapter 6.)

22. Inactivity

When was the last time you got out of the house and walked, jogged, or bicycled around the block? Or are you participating in any type of regular, moderate form of exertion? It's time to get up out of that chair and get active! Regular exercise is one of the best ways to maintain good health and condition the heart and prevent cardiovascular disease. Regular aerobic exercise helps raise the HDL levels, which helps remove plaque from the arteries in a process called *reversed cholesterol transport*. Exercise pumps oxygen to your cells, giving your body added ability to win the war against heart disease. Of course, any exercise program should be under the supervision of your doctor or health professional. The American College of Sports Medicine recommends a medical examination and exercise testing prior to participation in vigorous exercise for all males over forty-five and all females over fifty-five.

The average heart rate of an unconditioned heart at rest is about seventy-five to eighty-five beats per minute. A well-conditioned heart beats approximately sixty beats per minute. Since the unconditioned heart beats approximately twenty beats more per minute, that is an extra twelve hundred beats per hour, almost twenty-nine thousand extra beats per day, and over ten million extra beats per year!

Naturally, it would be great if your heart could do a little less work during your lifetime. The best way to lower your heart rate is to exercise regularly, for at least thirty minutes to an hour, four to five times per week. (For more information on exercise, please refer to my book *Get Fit and Live!*)

23. Gum disease

In 1998, the American Academy of Periodontology issued a statement that gum infections present a "far more dangerous threat" to the health of individuals than was previously thought. The reason is that gum infections caused by bacteria inspire inflammation not just in the mouth but also throughout the entire body and therefore increase the risks of cardiovascular disease and other complications. This means regular visits to your dentist may be as important as annual checkups with your doctor if you want to protect yourself from heart disease.

Periodontal bacteria can enter the bloodstream and invade arteries, causing the immune system to respond by producing antibodies against them. This increased level of antibodies can also inadvertently damage arteries and contribute to blood clots and plaque formation. In a fourteen-year study of ten thousand people between twenty-five and seventy-four years of age, it showed that subjects with great dental health suffered only a 10 percent incidence of cardiovascular disease, while if they had gingivitis, the risk went up to 14 percent. Those with periodontitis were 32 percent more likely to suffer CVD, and if a person's teeth had to be removed, they were 42 percent more likely to have CVD![16]

So, if you have missing or loose teeth, soft pus pockets in your mouth, even constant foul breath, you probably need to see your dentist as soon as possible. Other than that, every person should make regular trips to the dentist for cleaning and checkups—if nothing else, your heart health may well depend on this often overlooked risk factor.

24. Elevated ferritin level

Excessive iron contributes to cardiovascular disease because excess iron promotes inflammation and increases oxidized LDL cholesterol. It is also toxic to the endothelial cells, which line the arteries. Women who are menstruating lose blood as well as a significant amount of iron in the blood each month. But it's interesting that postmenopausal women are four times more likely to have heart attacks than premenopausal women. Low estrogen levels are a factor in this, but excessive iron is also another factor in causing cardiovascular disease. A Finnish study found that those with ferritin levels above 200 mcg/L were over twice as likely to have a heart attack.[17] An elevated ferritin level with an elevated cholesterol level increased the risk of heart attack to a fivefold greater risk. The ferritin level is a measure of your iron stores, and if it is elevated, you have excess iron in your body. If you are a male or a postmenopausal woman, do not take an iron supplement, even if the iron is in a multivitamin, unless you have a low ferritin level or you have iron deficiency. Then have your ferritin and CBC (complete blood count) checked periodically and go off the iron supplement as soon as the ferritin level is normal. Premenopausal women may take a multivitamin with iron if desired, but make sure you have your ferritin level checked yearly.

BETTER INFORMATION MAKES
FOR A BETTER FUTURE

Altogether this may seem overwhelming, but here's the good news: my experience in medicine tells me that no matter what condition your heart is in today, there is hope for health and recovery—yes, even if your parents or grandparents suffered from heart disease. If you'll simply follow the list of recommendations in this chapter, you will discover that clogged arteries can often be reversed without surgery. And remember God's Word with regard to everything I'm saying. Health and healing are what the Lord has in mind for you, just as He told the prophet long ago:

> "I will give you back your health and heal your wounds," says the LORD.
>
> —JEREMIAH 30:17

Of course, if you are indeed serious about reversing or preventing heart disease, you'll have to change the way you eat, give your body the supplements it needs, exercise regularly, and guard your thoughts. But don't try to change your lifestyle completely all at once. Just take some new steps every day, day by day, to a healthier heart.

A BIBLE CURE Prayer for You

Dear Jesus, just as You can give me a new heart spiritually, help me to strengthen and care for my natural heart by taking healthy, preventive steps through diet, nutrition, supplements, and exercise. Through Your Spirit, help me to be wise in implementing the knowledge that You have provided through Your grace. Amen.

A **BIBLE CURE** *Prescription*

Write a list of all the risk factors you need God to help you overcome and at least one thing you will begin to do today to overcome each item.

1. _____

2. _____

3. _____

4. _____

5. _____

6. _____

7. _____

Now, go back through this list, and thank God ahead of time for His help. When your prayer for help is answered, draw a line through the need and record the date you received your answer. You may be delightfully surprised to see how faithful God really is. This will prove a wonderful record of the goodness of God in your life.

4

CHELATION THERAPY

N 1956 DR. Norman Clarke was treating a battery worker for lead poisoning using ethylenediaminetetraacetic acid (EDTA). After the patient had finished his treatment, the doctor noticed that the man's angina had also disappeared. Soon other doctors began following in Dr. Clarke's footsteps, and in 1972 the American College for the Advancement of Medicine was formed in order to educate physicians and to provide additional research for chelation therapy.[1]

> I know how to live on almost nothing or with everything. I have learned the secret of living in every situation, whether it is with a full stomach or empty, with plenty or little. For I can do everything through Christ, who gives me strength.
> —PHILIPPIANS 4:12–13

Chelation therapy uses EDTA along with vitamins and minerals to improve blood flow and to chelate and purge the body of toxic heavy metals. Initially it was thought that EDTA unclogged arteries by removing the calcium out of the plaque. We now know that it improves blood flow by removing iron, copper, lead, cadmium, and other toxic metals from the body.

Doctors who administer chelation therapy recognize that atherosclerosis not only affects the arteries of the heart but also the smallest arteries and capillaries in the fingers, toes, brain, and throughout the entire body. In other words, the therapy improves blood flow throughout the entire body, whereas angioplasties and coronary bypass grafts only treat small areas of atherosclerosis.

Patients suffering from atherosclerosis and lead poisoning have reported surprising benefits from chelation. These benefits included: (1) patients were able to walk farther; (2) patients with angina were able to exercise more strenuously without developing chest pain; and (3) patients with leg pain from poor circulation many times no longer experienced pain or were able to walk farther before leg pain developed. Along with these symptom-reducing benefits is the fact that EDTA also restores the normal production of prostacyclin, the prostaglandin hormone that prevents blood clots and arterial spasms and improves blood flow, even in diseased arteries.

EDTA can also reduce the production of free radicals, which attack our cell structures and weaken our immune systems by as much as a millionfold! I believe that anyone with poor circulation, along with heavy metal toxicity (such as cadmium and lead poisoning) should consider having chelation therapy at least one time per week for twenty to forty treatments and then continue chelation therapy once a month as maintenance.[2]

CHELATION THERAPY

There are diverse opinions about chelation therapy. Here is the official statement of the American Heart Association concerning chelation therapy as posted at their Web site at www.americanheart.org in 2010.

> Chelation therapy is administering a man-made amino acid called EDTA into the veins. (EDTA is an abbreviation for ethylenediaminetetraacetic acid. It's marketed under several names, including Edetate, Disodium, Endrate, and Sodium Versenate.) EDTA is most often used in cases of heavy metal poisoning (lead or mercury). That's because it can latch onto or bind these metals, creating a compound that can be excreted in the urine.
>
> Besides binding heavy metals, EDTA also "chelates" (naturally seeks out and binds) calcium, one of the components of atherosclerotic plaque. In the early 1960s, this led to speculation that EDTA could remove calcium deposits from buildups in arteries. The idea was that once the calcium was removed by regular treatments of EDTA, the remaining elements in the plaque would break up and the plaque would clear away. The narrowed arteries would be restored to their former state.
>
> Based upon this thinking, chelation therapy has been proposed to treat existing atherosclerosis and to prevent it from forming.
>
> After carefully reviewing all the available scientific literature on this subject, the American Heart Association has concluded that the benefits claimed for this form of therapy aren't scientifically proven.

That's why we don't recommend this type of treatment.[3]

There are, however, multitudes of individual testimonies that support that this therapy has benefits for those suffering from heavy metal toxicity and cardiovascular disease. If you are considering chelation therapy, I would encourage you to do your own research on chelation therapy and draw your own conclusion as to what would be best for you. If you have heavy metal toxicity, such as excessive amounts of lead, cadmium, or mercury on a six-hour urine test after taking a chelation agent such as DMSA or EDTA, then you would probably benefit from chelation therapy. Recall that practically everyone on Planet Earth has lead stored in their body with approximately 90 percent of the lead in the body being in the bones. After menopause when bone loss accelerates in women, so does their risk of osteoporosis and heart disease, but realize that lead is also being released from their bones as they demineralize. A similar scenario occurs in men, but bone loss is usually slower in men. An individual's lead content is directly associated with an increased risk of hypertension and cardiovascular disease.

TRIAL TO ASSESS CHELATION THERAPY (TACT)

The National Institutes of Health (NIH) began the TACT study, or Trial to Assess Chelation Therapy, in August 2002. This is the first large study to determine whether EDTA chelation therapy is safe and effective for patients with coronary artery disease. This trial uses sodium EDTA that requires approximately four hours treatment. The TACT study should determine whether individuals who have chelation therapy and take an oral vitamin and mineral supplement during the five years will have fewer heart attacks and fewer cardiac surgeries or stents. The results will be available December 2011.

A **BIBLE CURE** Prayer for You

Almighty God, heal my body and remove the pain of angina. I speak to my heart and entire circulatory system to be healed in Jesus's name. Lord, I ask for Your guidance in the right steps to take to remove plaque from my arteries and to live by faith, not doubt; by hope, not discouragement; and to live in divine health, not sickness, in Jesus's name. Amen.

A **BIBLE CURE** *Prescription*

Do you have heavy metal toxicity? Do you have numerous silver fillings? Do you have elevated levels of lead, cadmium, or mercury on either a hair analysis or a six-hour urine test for toxic metals after a challenge? To find a doctor who can help you with these questions, see appendix.

Write a prayer, using your own words, asking God for His wisdom and help as you consider your treatment options:

_____

_____

_____

_____

_____

NUTRITIONAL SUPPLEMENTS FOR CONGESTIVE HEART FAILURE AND ARRHYTHMIA

ACCORDING TO THE American Heart Association, congestive heart failure—often just called heart failure—affects roughly 5.7 million Americans and is diagnosed in another 670,000 each year. It is characterized by a weakening of the heart muscle that decreases its ability to pump blood effectively, usually because oxygen and nutrients are slowly cut off to it over time because of the reduced blood flow caused by atherosclerosis. While congestive heart failure can be fatal, it is also treatable and can be controlled—sometimes even reversed—with the proper care, lifestyle changes, and supplements.

Arrhythmia is another heart complication that affects millions of Americans. An arrhythmia is an abnormality in the rhythm of the heartbeat. A healthy heart may experience this from time to time, but consistent problems with arrhythmia may be a sign of a more severe problem with your heart. This will also make the heart less effective in pumping blood to all the parts of the body that need the crucial oxygen and nutrients it carries and may be associated with congestive heart failure.

The heart is the most specialized muscle in the body having only one responsibility, to keep blood flowing throughout the entire 60,000-mile pipeline that is the cardiovascular system. It does this twenty-four hours a day, day-in and day-out, while we sleep, sit, exercise, or whatever else we do in the course of our days. To do this it needs constant oxygen and nutrition to carry out its function without coffee breaks, weekends off, changes in its work patterns, or naps.

A healthy heart will pump out 50 to 70 percent of the blood in it (called the "ejection fraction" or EF) with each contraction or beat. As the heart ages, especially if anything interferes with the flow of oxygen and sugar to feed it, the EF will begin to drop. A heart is considered to be failing when the EF with each contraction reaches 40 percent or less. This then becomes a downward spiral as other parts of the body also slowly starve from lack of oxygen and important nutrients. This may also cause fluid to back up in the lungs, causing congestion (the "congestive" part of congestive heart failure). CHF can be considered mild, average, severe, or very severe depending on how much the heart is failing.

One of the first signs of congestive heart failure is often weight gain as fluid starts to collect in the abdomen, feet, ankles, and legs. The person may also feel tired more easily or have a shortness of breath when doing what would otherwise be a mild increase in exertion—climbing stairs or after a brisk walk to catch a bus. They may wake up with a choking sensation as they experience shortness of breath because their lungs are filling with fluid. If this worsens, it will lead to a persistent cough that may even contain mucus or even blood. They may also experience angina symptoms. Anyone experiencing such symptoms should consult a physician immediately.

Arrhythmia, on the other hand, may have no outward symptoms at all and may only be detected by a doctor with a stethoscope or through an electrocardiogram. However, others may experience heart palpitations (any of the irregularities of the heartbeat as mentioned above), dizziness or light-headedness, a "pounding" chest, fainting or shortness of breath, unusual fatigue or weakness, or general chest discomfort. Again, if you experience something like this, see your physician right away or go to the ER.

While the heart ages just as we do, such problems do not normally manifest without additional complications. High blood pressure will eventually make the heart work harder than it should and put more wear and tear on it than is needed. This will eventually lead to its "tiring" or "misfiring." Narrowing of the arteries will limit the oxygen and nutrients to the heart, slowly starving it. Heart attacks can damage parts of the heart that may never recover, thus weakening the heart. The heart may also get infected or attacked by disease, a condition called cardiomyopathy. Other conditions that can gradually weaken the heart are diabetes, cancer treatments, thyroid problems, alcohol and drug abuse, as well as other serious, less common ailments. Congestive heart failure is most common in people over sixty-five, men, and African Americans. The dangers of arrhythmia also increase with age.

HOPE FOR CONGESTIVE HEART FAILURE AND ARRHYTHMIA

While congestive heart failure is very serious and certain arrhythmias could lead to sudden death, they are typically both very treatable. As with most muscles in the body, the heart can be maintained and even strengthened. Treatment is all about reenergizing and refueling the heart by increasing blood flow to it and supplying nutrients to strengthen the heart and give it more energy. You might think of it like recharging the "battery cells" of the heart. It is really a question of getting as much "energy" generated for the heart as possible.

As with any other muscle, this energy starts at the cellular level, and the powerhouse of the cell is mitochondria, small organelles inside of each cell that generate energy by synthesizing fuel (food) and oxygen and making ATP. Mitochondria generate over 90 percent of the energy the body uses and make up about 35 percent of heart cells. It is mitochondrial energy that drives the metabolism. ATP is the heart's energy currency. Mitochondrial energy is produced in a process that uses oxygen and nutrients to change adenosine triphosphate (ATP) into adenosine diphosphate (ADP) and inorganic phosphate (P_i), then changes those two back to ATP again. This cycle is almost like the turning of a turbine, releasing energy with each change. If the cell is deficient in fuel or oxygen, this cycle suffers; thus the cell's metabolism suffers and its function is compromised.

The by-product of this cycle is carbon dioxide (CO_2), water, and a small amount of damaged oxygen molecules that are missing an electron—in other words, free radicals. The CO_2 is exhaled when we breathe, along with a little of the water, while the rest of the water travels to the kidneys. If the free radicals accumulate to high levels, it can cause problems; however, there is evidence that some level of them may be important for functions such as mitochondrial respiration, white blood cell activity, and platelet activation. Very high levels, though, will injure the cell membranes, degrade the mitochondria and other parts of the cell, as well as damage DNA. To prevent this, I recommend glutathione-boosting supplements, which is the body's most important antioxidant. (See appendix.)

The key to optimizing this energy-producing cycle is keeping the mitochondria healthy. If we have healthy mitochondria, then we will be healthy too. Healthy mitochondria protect against any number of degenerative diseases like cardiovascular disease, cancer, and Alzheimer's disease.

NUTRIENTS FOR A HEALTHY HEART MUSCLE

Coenzyme Q_{10}: The antioxidant coenzyme Q_{10} (CoQ_{10}) functions as a coenzyme in the energy-producing pathways of every cell in the body and is an important antioxidant that will fight the oxidation that creates free radicals as well as the oxidation of LDL and other lipids. CoQ_{10} is found in many foods, such as broccoli, Chinese cabbage, spinach, raw nuts, ocean fish and shellfish, pork, chicken, and beef. However, in a normal diet, we only get 2–5 mg of this important vitamin-like compound, so it is wise to add it in supplement form as well.

CoQ_{10} is one of the best "electron donors" that gives its electrons freely to electron-deficient free radicals rendering them harmless. It also restores oxidized vitamin E into a useful form. By given electrons to vitamin E—which, as you recall, is another important antioxidant—it "recycles" vitamin E to get it back into the free radical fight once again. In this way, when supplements of vitamin E and CoQ_{10} are combined, LDL becomes more resistant to oxidation than when you take vitamin E alone. This combination has also been shown to reduce C-reactive protein (CRP) levels in laboratory animals. However, CoQ_{10}'s most important function is probably within the mitochondria that facilitate the cycle of ATP to ADP to ATP—and so on—which is so crucial to the health of every cell and particularly important in the cells of the heart muscle.

When you take CoQ_{10} as a supplement, pay attention to what form it comes in. Research has shown that since it is such a large molecule, it is hard to absorb. The best form to take it in is ubiquinol, which is the active form. As many as 30 percent of Japanese have a defective NQ01 gene that regulates coenzyme Q_{10} from the inactive ubiquinone to the active ubiquinol. Also, as you age, the conversion process slows down. For basic health, I recommend 100 mg of ubiquinol a day. For CHF I recommend ubiquinol 100 mg, three times a day, and for severe CHF you may need ubiquinol 200 mg, two to three times a day. If you are taking a statin drug, I recommend 100–300 mg a day of ubiquinol. I also check the CoQ_{10} blood level and adjust the dose accordingly. Life Extension performs this blood test.

L-carnitine: Another "transport" molecule that helps in mitochondrial energy generation is L-carnitine, which facilitates moving long-chain fatty acids across the inner mitochondrial membrane to catalyze beta-oxidation, a process by which the fat is broken down so it can be burned as fuel and turned into energy. L-carnitine is one of the most easily used amino acids in our bodies and is also a precursor of nitric oxide and other metabolites. These fatty acids must be brought through the mitochondrial membrane to be processed in this way, and L-carnitine is the only carrier molecule that can do this. Thus the higher the level of L-carnitine in your system, the greater the rate of energy metabolism, and the lower the level, the more difficult it is to generate sufficient energy. Since the heart gets at least 60 percent of its fuel from such fat sources, L-carnitine is crucial to heart health and improving congestive heart failure.

L-carnitine is found in protein-rich foods such as peanuts, Brazil nuts, walnuts, coconut, milk and milk products, pork, beef, chicken, turkey, seafood, oats, wheat, and chocolate. However, with age, through genetic defects or eating carnitine-deficient diets (such as pure vegetarians often do), deficiencies of other vitamins and minerals important to L-carnitine, liver or kidney disease, and the use of certain prescription drugs are all associated with our bodies having insufficient levels of L-carnitine; therefore, supplementation is vital. L-carnitine should be supplemented in a dose of 500 mg, three times a day. For severe CHF, I usually increase the dose to 1,000 mg, three times a day.

D-ribose is a simple five-carbon sugar found in every cell of the body. It is different from other sugars, such as glucose (a six-carbon sugar) because it both provides and sustains energy, especially in weakened hearts. D-ribose provides tremendous support to the mitochondria in assisting the mitochondria to produce ATP, or the heart's energy currency.

D-ribose is naturally present in some meats, but only in trace amounts so small it does not really make any meaningful impact on our bodies. Cells synthesize D-ribose as they need it to varying degrees, but supplementation of D-ribose is the best way to provide it within your body because it is easily absorbed and put to work.

I recommend the following daily dosages for the following concerns:

- As a daily preventative of cardiovascular disease
  or those who exercise strenuously on a regular

basis: 5–7 g a day (5 g is equivalent to 2 teaspoons)

- For someone with mild to moderate congestive heart failure, recovering from a heart attack or heart surgery, treatment of angina, or those with other significant vascular concerns: 7–10 g a day in divided doses

- For advanced congestive heart failure, dilated cardiomyopathy, frequent angina, and those awaiting heart transplants or suffering from fibromyalgia: 10–15 g a day in divided doses (see appendix)

Magnesium is a wonderful mineral for the heart and cardiovascular system across the board. If you're suffering with congestive heart failure or arrhythmia, magnesium should be a significant help to you. In fact, magnesium deficiency is very common in those who have congestive heart failure. Studies show that as many as half of Americans lack the magnesium they should have, oddly enough roughly the same number that have cardiovascular complications.

Magnesium is present in nuts, grains, beans, and dark green vegetables. Alcohol and caffeine consumption encourage the excretion of magnesium. Certain conventional drugs for treating congestive heart failure, such as Lanoxin and various diuretics, may also deplete magnesium levels.

All individuals who have experienced congestive heart failure should take a magnesium supplement. It is also beneficial in treating arrhythmia, including atrial fibrillation, PVCs, and symptoms of mitral valve prolapse. I recommend a dose of 200 mg, two to three times a day. Use caution with magnesium since it may cause diarrhea. Start with 200 mg and increase very slowly if needed.

Testosterone supplementation is also very important for all people with CHF. There are more testosterone receptors in cardiac muscle than any other muscles in the body. Testosterone will also help strengthen the heart muscle. I even place women with CHF on testosterone, usually with a 2–5 mg lozenge once a day. Heavy metal detoxification, chelation therapy, and an infrared sauna are also very important for people with CHF. People with CHF many times have very high mercury, lead, and/or cadmium levels in their cardiac muscle, and their heavy metals are poisoning their mitochondria or their energy-producing structures in the cell. I also recommend omega-3 fats and glutathione-boosting supplements for patients with congestive heart failure.

ARRHYTHMIA

The above supplements not only help CHF but also help arrhythmia. An arrhythmia is any change in the regular rhythm of the heart. It is typically due to interference with the electrical pathways of the heart and are responsible for over 400,000 deaths each year. Some arrhythmias are harmless and some are life threatening. Often the first sign of hidden heart disease is sudden death, which is usually caused by arrhythmias.

Omega-3 fats

Omega-3 fats from fish oil may prevent sudden death. The Italian GISSI-Prevenzione was a trial of over eleven thousand participants who either took 1,000 mg of EPA and DHA (fish oil) or a placebo. The group taking fish oil had a 30 percent reduction in cardiovascular mortality and a 45 percent reduction in sudden death.[1] A Harvard study showed that men who had higher blood levels of omega-3 fats had an 80 percent lower risk of sudden death compared with men with low serum levels of omega-3.[2] Omega-3 fats may also help prevent atrial fibrillation. (See appendix.)

Magnesium

Magnesium deficiency is associated with arrhythmias including atrial fibrillation and atrial flutter. Atrial fibrillation is the most common sustained arrhythmia. Magnesium strongly impacts heart cell membrane function and is a very important catalyst in many enzymatic reactions in the heart muscle cell (myocyte) and in more than three hundred enzymatic reactions in the body. Magnesium given by intravenously has also been shown to reduce the frequency of ventricular arrhythmias in patients with symptomatic heart failure. Magnesium helps to prevent both benign arrhythmias and serious arrhythmias. Magnesium helps to relax the heart and calm down and stabilize the heart's electrical system. I typically recommend 200 mg of chelated magnesium two to three times a day. Start with a low dose and increase slowly to prevent diarrhea. (See appendix.)

Taurine

Taurine is the second most abundant amino acid in muscle. Foods that contain taurine include meat, poultry, eggs, dairy, and fish. Taurine prevents arrhythmias by limiting calcium overload of the myocardium and helping to prevent hypertrophy of the heart. The heart that is ischemic or lacking adequate oxygen is more prone to arrhythmia. Some researchers believe that arrhythmias due to acute myocardial ischemic may be due to a loss of intracellular taurine. Following either an ischemic event or heart attack, taurine levels drop to as low as one-third of normal levels. Taurine also protects the oxygen-starved, or ischemic, heart from reperfusion-induced arrhythmias. I recommend at least 500–1,000 mg twice a day; however, doses up to 6,000 mg a day have been used in some studies.

Coenzyme Q_{10} (ubiquinol)

I have already discussed CoQ_{10} in detail; however, it is also very useful in treating arrhythmias. CoQ_{10} is found in every cell of the body and helps manufacture energy. It also is believed to stabilize the heart's electrical system and help prevent arrhythmias. It is especially effective for PVCs, or premature ventricular contractions. I usually recommend ubiquinol in a daily dose of 100–300 mg a day.

Berberine

Berberine is the main active ingredient in the herb goldenseal, which has been used for years to treat intestinal infections. It has also been found to be beneficial for ventricular arrhythmias due to ischemia or a lack of oxygen. Berberine may also help prevent sudden death after myocardial ischemic damage. Researchers have studied berberine on patients with ventricular arrhythmias. They found that 62 percent of patients had 50 percent or greater, and 38 percent of patients had 90 percent or greater suppression of PVC, or premature ventricular contractions. Berberine is typically recommended at a dose of 500 mg, twice a day.

Most all supplements that help congestive heart failure and ischemia will also typically help arrhythmias. Therefore, refer to prior sections of the book. Also the herb hawthorn can help control benign arrhythmias in a dose of 80–300 mg twice a day.

FINALLY, A BETTER WAY TO LIVE

In 1 Corinthians 15:31, the apostle Paul said, "I face death daily." In effect, Paul was living what many call the "crucified life." It's a way of approaching each day in peace, knowing that our lives and futures are in God's hands, knowing that we have let Him have our egos and everything else that ought to matter so much less to us than God's kingdom. I highly recommend this way of living. It's good for the heart, and it's good for the soul.

The most wonderful thing about the crucified life is that we can make it our own at any moment. We simply choose to adjust our focus. In the face of potential stress, imminent worry, or intruding anxiety, we can remind ourselves:

> My old self has been crucified with Christ. It is no longer I who live, but Christ lives in me. So I live in this earthly body by trusting in the Son of God, who loved me and gave himself for me.
>
> —GALATIANS 2:20

Ultimately, being in God's hands and following His ways for how to live and be healthy is the best place to be. Pray over these things, and ask His guidance for how best to follow His and your doctor's advice. Neither congestive heart failure nor arrhythmia are God's best for you. He has a better plan for fullness through the wisdom He has already put in the earth for your healing. Don't let a day go by that you are not pursuing Him for His best for you and your heart.

A **BIBLE CURE** *for You*

Dear Lord, thank You for creating my body as a complex,
powerful, wonderful living being. Moreover, thank You
for providing wisdom and understanding to help me
release the healing virtue You have already placed within
my body. Provide me with all the insight I need to begin
walking in Your wonderful divine health. Amen.

A **BIBLE CURE** Prescription

Recap Your Progress

In light of all you've learned, list three things you are NOT doing now that you need to do to lower the risk of heart disease in your future:

1. _____

2. _____

3. _____

List three things you ARE doing right that you need to keep doing:

1. _____

2. _____

3. _____

Jot down three Scripture passages that build hope in you as you overcome heart disease:

1. _____

2. _____

3. _____

OTHER WAYS TO TRACK YOUR ARTERIAL PLAQUE

O NCE YOU REACH the age of forty, annual physicals (before the age of forty I recommend physicals every two years) are a first line of detection for risk factors of cardiovascular and other life-threatening diseases. Typically your doctor will give you a standard battery of tests designed to look for factors that may put you at risk for cardiovascular disease down the road. Unfortunately, most doctors do not perform a comprehensive test that looks at numerous potential markers of heart disease.

CORONARY COMPUTERIZED TOMOGRAPHY (CT) SCANS

New methods and procedures are being discovered and experimented with constantly to find better ways of predicting the true threats of cardiovascular disease suddenly ending an individual's life with a heart attack or sudden death. While standard blood tests give us feedback on the presence of certain risk factors, they do not give us a very good picture of how much buildup is already taking place within arteries, how blood flow is being affected, and how many potential "hot spots" are present where plaque might rupture to cause a sudden ischemic event. Thus more and more doctors are letting their patients know about such examinations as the coronary CT scan.

A computerized tomography (CT or CAT) scan is done by taking a number of CT "slices" of a person's body and internal organs from various angles and then reassembling them with a computer into a three-dimensional image of the organ(s) concerned. The procedure is noninvasive (meaning they don't have to put anything into your body), though it does carry some risk because of the higher radiation level than would happen with standard X-rays (approximately equal to one hundred fifty chest X-rays). These risks, however, are usually outweighed by the valuable information the examination gives the patient. I do not recommend these tests too frequently (not more than once every one to two years) due to the radiation you can receive.

A **BIBLE CURE** Health Fact

What Your Coronary CT Scan Score Means

Calcium Score	Amount of calcified plaque	Chance of blockage in the foreseeable future
0	None	Highly unlikely
1–10	Minimal	Highly unlikely
11–100	Mild	Low likelihood
101–400	Moderate	11–25% likelihood
Over 400	Extensive	More than 50% likelihood

When this is done specifically to detect coronary heart disease, the CT scan will give feedback on the presence, location, and amount of calcified plaque in the arteries. The findings can then be easily turned into a *calcium score* that indicates the amount of plaque that has accumulated as well as a means to monitor your plaque reversal. This calcium score will also help predict the likelihood of a cardiovascular incident happening in your future.

Some of the limitations of this exam are that for people under the age of fifty, their atherosclerosis may not yet have calcified enough to be detected by a CT scan; however, new CT scan software is able to detect soft plaque that is not yet calcified. Also, very few health insurance companies cover this exam at this writing. And for any given calcium score, there is not yet a prescribed line of treatment to specifically address that level of risk. Nor can a specific number tell you just how much blockage you have at present, only the statistical likelihood of it being present. On the other hand, any amount of plaque can lead to a rupture and a heart attack; however, unstable plaque is more likely to rupture compared to stable plaque. You may have a high calcium score that indicates significant plaque; however, if the inflammation is controlled as indicated by a low CRP and low LP PLA2 test, the plaque is stable and significantly less likely to rupture.

While cholesterol tests will give you a snapshot of your current diet and lifestyle, it will not give you a cumulative total of how your past lifestyle might still be affecting you today. A CT scan, on the other hand, will. No matter what you are doing today, a CT scan will show the cumulative effects of your lifetime's lifestyle in how much plaque has built up over your years, and thus it gives you a much better picture of your actual risk than standard blood tests will.

If you want to significantly increase the probability that you will stabilize and reduce your plaque, you should do what you need to in order to lower your LDL number below 70 and raise your HDL number above 60, as well as lower the CRP and PL PLA2 numbers to normal. Review the pertinent sections in chapter 3 for strategies to do this, and then discuss them with your doctor. Also ,have all risk factors checked and modified by following the strategies outlined in this book. Have all positive risk factors rechecked until they are in normal range.

CAROTID ULTRASOUND IMT SCORE

Not surprisingly perhaps, the health of the carotid arteries (the ones that carry oxygen and nutrients to the brain) can give great insight into the health of the cardiovascular system overall. It is also a quick, noninvasive, and easy measurement to take and without radiation.

The exam determines the thickness of the artery wall and compares the ratio of the endothelium (the thin, innermost layer of a blood vessel) to the medial (or middle layer). This will give you an Intema Media Thickness Score, which will tell you the amount of plaque in your carotid artery and which will indirectly give you an indication of what the plaque is probably like in the rest of your arteries and more directly what your risk is of experiencing a stroke. It is noninvasive and requires no X-ray and can be used to track your plaque. It is also covered by most insurance companies.

GENOVA DIAGNOSTICS CARDIOVASCULAR HEALTH PLUS GENOMICS

This comprehensive blood test analyzes lipid markers and advanced markers for cardiovascular disease as well as a patient's genomic predisposition to cardiovascular disease. It includes the genomic markers APOE, MTHFR (the enzyme in folate metabolism), and Factor II and Factor V (causes increased risk of blood clots). Advanced markers include LDL-particle number, HDL-particle number, LDL-size, hs-CRP, Lp(a), Lp-PLA2, homocysteine level, fibrinogen level, and insulin resistance score. This is a very economical test that gives a tremendous amount of information that by modifying the risk factors, can save your life. (See appendix.)

The Berkeley Heartlab

This is the most comprehensive cardiac panel I have seen, but it is rather expensive. It includes LDL particle size as a distribution of seven subclasses, HDL particle size as a distribution of five subclasses, Apo B, Lp(a), homocysteine, APOE, LPA aspirin check genotype test, statin check genotype test, Lp-PLA2, hs-CRP, insulin, WT-pro BWP (detection of clinical and subclinical cardiac dysfunction), and Q-LDL (atherogenic subclass of ventilation). The Berkeley Heartlab is an excellent test and also offers a 4MyHeart program for disease management. (See appendix.)

THE VERTICAL AUTO PROFILE (VAP)

A vertical auto profile is a more thorough test for different types of cholesterol. While it tests LDL and HDL levels, it also breaks these down further into subcategories that research is finding have greater value. For instance, they test for two forms of HDL cholesterol, commonly referred to as HDL1 and HDL2, of which HDL2 is the more important to cardiovascular health. In others words, a high HDL count in a normal cholesterol test could be slightly misleading if it was mostly HDL1, or a low HDL level could be better if it was almost all HDL2. It also tests LDL subcategories and for Lp(a) levels. The VAP uses a blood sample just as standard blood tests do, even though the feedback is much more specific. (See appendix.)

NMR LIPOPROFILE

The NMR Lipoprofile uses a nuclear magnetic resonance (NMR) spectroscopy to give a quick, snapshot measurement of the size and number of LDL particles as well those of HDL and VLDL (very-low-density lipoproteins). This information allows doctors and patients to design more specific treatment programs than standard cholesterol tests. As we have already seen, it is not the level of overall LDL that is dangerous as much as it is the number of LDL particles. Also, VLDL particles have been shown to be just as dangerous if not more dangerous than simple LDL because they have a tendency to increase the number of LDL clusters and weaken the effectiveness of HDL particles. Thankfully, VLDL responds to many of the same interventions as triglycerides and LDL do. (See appendix.)

MORE INFORMATION, BETTER TREATMENT!

I realize that so much information can seem overwhelming, but I don't share it in order to discourage you. I want you to be better informed so that you can be better able to live the life God has planned for you from the beginning. Whatever your situation, remember that your life, with all its joys and sorrows, is always held close to God's own heart. Your heart matters to His! So trust in His goodness for today, tomorrow, and each day thereafter. He cares for you, and His promise is never to leave you. (See Matthew 28:20.) That is the greatest promise you could ever have, and it will see you though whatever challenges—including facing cardiovascular disease—that life on this earth could ever throw at you.

> Let your face smile on us, LORD. You have given me greater joy than those who have abundant harvests of grain and new wine. In peace I will lie down and sleep, for you alone, O LORD, will keep me safe.
> —PSALM 4:6–8

A BIBLE CURE *Prayer for You*

Dear Lord, I cast all my care, concern, worry, fear, and lack of control upon You. Let me exchange my weakness for Your power, my fear for Your courage, and my lack for Your control. I receive Your healing touch. Amen.

A **BIBLE CURE** Prescription

Marking Time With God

It's time to stop thinking about medicine for a little while! In a few minutes of silence, turn your thoughts to the Lord and meditate upon each verse below. When you're through, remain still and quiet before the Lord; consider your responses in His presence. How do they reveal the true desires of your heart? Your most pressing needs? Your greatest challenges as you confront heart disease? Simply underline the phrases that most apply to your situation and then pray, asking God to meet your needs and heal your body.

Read each verse:

Isaiah 41:10
1 Peter 5:10–11
Philippians 3:20–21

If possible, during the coming week, share your scripture markings with a family member, friend, or pastor. Talk about them together, and then encourage one another.

YOUR HEART DISEASE PREVENTION PLAN

I N CLOSING, LET me remind you that when you eat the right things and stop eating the wrong things, you are contributing to your health in more ways than one. You are also strengthening the life of the Spirit within you through your honoring of the One who "owns" you.

> Don't you realize that your body is the temple of the Holy Spirit, who lives in you and was given to you by God? You do not belong to yourself, for God bought you with a high price. So you must honor God with your body.
>
> —1 CORINTHIANS 6:19–20

THE GREATEST MEDICINE

All of these natural approaches will benefit you greatly. But what will benefit you the most is your faith in God. He is a wonderful Creator of limitless power and imagination. Yet He loves you more deeply than you could ever imagine. Don't ever think your health does not matter to Him. Everything about you matters to Him! The Bible says that He has even counted the number of hairs on your head! (See Luke 12:7.) He cares deeply about every miniscule detail in your life—and His power is beyond your comprehension. Begin to speak His blessings and claim His healing.

> Let all that I am praise the LORD; with my whole heart, I will praise his holy name. Let all that I am praise the LORD; may I never forget the good things he does for me. He forgives all my sins and heals all my diseases. He redeems me from death and crowns me with love and tender mercies. He fills my life with good things. My youth is renewed like the eagle's!
>
> —PSALM 103:1–5

> We are pressed on every side by troubles, but we are not crushed. We are perplexed, but not driven to despair. We are hunted down, but never abandoned by God. We get knocked down, but we are not destroyed. Through suffering, our bodies continue to share in the death of Jesus so that the life of Jesus may also be seen in our bodies.
>
> —2 CORINTHIANS 4:8–10

Now, if you are trying the nutrients I've mentioned in the previous pages and maintaining your close fellowship with the Lord, you might also think about another kind of therapy for keeping your heart healthy.

Are You Looking Ahead?

As we have seen, the foundational problem for almost all heart disease is poor coronary artery circulation due to atherosclerosis. Atherosclerosis also may cause a diminished blood supply to vital organs of the body, including the brain, heart, and kidneys. Poor blood supply, in turn, causes more plaque to form, which creates a vicious cycle that may well eventually lead to heart attack, stroke, kidney failure, or the possible amputation of an extremity.

God knows the pain you feel from the diseases and has given you both spiritual and natural ways to end cardiovascular disease and walk in divine health. It's now up to you to step out in faith and apply the knowledge you have. As you jot down your particular Bible cure prescription, remember His healing promise: "But he was pierced for our rebellion, crushed for our sins. He was beaten so we could be whole. He was whipped so we could be healed" (Isa. 53:5).

Keeping the Blessing

Anyone who loses his good health will tell you that it is a precious gift from God. Too many of us are guilty of squandering this treasure by not caring for our health the way that we should. When it's gone, we live with regrets. How much better to make healthy lifestyle choices before we lose our good health?

The English writer Izaak Walton once wrote, "Look to your health; and if you have it, praise God, and value it next to a good conscience." He also said that health is a blessing from God that money cannot buy. It's true. All the money in the world usually cannot replace your good health once you have lost it. Be grateful for the gift of good health that you have, and renew your commitment to keep it. It is a precious treasure!

> Through the power of the Holy Spirit who lives within us, carefully guard the precious truth that has been entrusted to you.
>
> —2 TIMOTHY 1:14

A Personal Note

FROM DON COLBERT

G OD DESIRES TO heal you of disease. His Word is full of promises that confirm His love for you and His desire to give you His abundant life. His desire includes more than physical health for you; He wants to make you whole in your mind and spirit as well through a personal relationship with His Son, Jesus Christ.

If you haven't met my best friend, Jesus, I would like to take this opportunity to introduce Him to you. It is very simple. If you are ready to let Him come into your life and become your best friend, all you need to do is sincerely pray this prayer:

> *Lord Jesus, I want to know You as my Savior and Lord. I believe You are the Son of God and that You died for my sins. I also believe You were raised from the dead and now sit at the right hand of the Father praying for me. I ask You to forgive me for my sins and change my heart so that I can be Your child and live with You eternally. Thank You for Your peace. Help me to walk with You so that I can begin to know You as my best friend and my Lord. Amen.*

If you have prayed this prayer, you have just made the most important decision of your life. I rejoice with you in your decision and your new relationship with Jesus. Please contact my publisher at pray4me@strang.com so that we can send you some materials that will help you become established in your relationship with the Lord. We look forward to hearing from you.

APPENDIX

Supplements are listed in alphabetical order.

Berkeley Heartlab—www.bhlinc.com

Bioidentical HRT—www.worldhealth.net

Chelation therapy—call 1-800-LEADOUT

Coenzyme Q_{10} (ubiquinol)—Living CoQ_{10}; available at www.drcolbert.com

D-ribose—Corvalen; available at www.drcolbert.com

Fish oil—Living Omega; available at www.drcolbert.com

Folic acid (active form)—FolaPro; available at www.drcolbert.meta-ehealth.com. Use code w7741.

Genomic testing—available at www.drcolbert.com

Genova—www.gdx.net

Glutathione-boosting supplement—Max GXL; available at www.max.com. Use distribution #231599.

Irvingia—available at www.drcolbert.com

L-arginine and L-citrulline—ProArgi-9; available from www.drcolbert.mysynergy.net

Magnesium—Chelated Magnesium; available at www.drcolbert.com

Multivitamin—Divine Health Multivitamin, Living Multivitamin; available at www.drcolbert.com

Nattokinase—available from www.drcolbert.com

Niacin—available from www.drcolbert.com

NMR Lipoprofile—www.liposcience.com

Pine bark and grape seed extract—OPCs; available at www.drcolbert.com

Plant sterols—Cardio-Edge; available from www.drcolbert.com

Red yeast rice—LipiControl; available from www.drcolbert.com

Resveratrol and quercetin—Living Resveratrol; available at www.drcolbert.com

Soluble fiber—PGX fiber; available at www.drcolbert.com

Vertical Auto Profile (VAP)—www.vaptest.com

Zeolites—Natural Cellular Defense; available at www.mywaiora.com

NOTES

INTRODUCTION
A NEW BIBLE CURE WITH NEW HOPE FOR YOUR HEART

1. American Heart Association, *Heart Disease and Stroke Statistics—2010 Update* (Dallas, Texas: American Heart Association, 2010), http://www.americanheart .org/downloadable/heart/1265665152970DS-3241 %20HeartStrokeUpdate_2010.pdf (accessed February 23, 2010).

2. American Heart Association, "Cardiovascular Disease Statistics," http://www.americanheart.org/presenter .jhtml?identifier=4478 (accessed April 14, 2010).

CHAPTER 1
HOPE TO BEAT THE STATISTICS FOR HEART DISEASE

1. American Heart Association, "Heart, How It Works," http:// www.americanheart.org/presenter.jhtml?identifier=4642 (accessed April 14, 2010).

2. American Heart Association, "Cardiovascular Disease Statistics."

3. American Heart Association, *Heart Disease and Stroke Statistics—2010 Update.*

4. "Diagonal Earlobe Creases and Prognosis in Patients With Suspected Coronary Artery Disease," *American Medical Journal* 100 (1996): 205–211.

5. Dean Haycock, "Are Balding Men at Risk?" WebMD Feature, July 27, 2001, http://www.medicinenet.com/script/main/art. asp?articlekey=51027 (accessed June 21, 2010).

CHAPTER 2
INFLAMMATION: THE ROOT CAUSE OF HEART DISEASE

1. "Heart Attack," Heart Online, http://www.heartonline.org/heart_attack.htm (accessed March 19, 2010).

2. H. C. McGill et al., "Association of Coronary Heart Disease Risk Factors With Microscopic Qualities of Coronary Atherosclerosis in Youth," *Circulation* 102 (2000): 374–379.

3. William Davis, "New Blood Test Better Predicts Heart Attack Risk," *Life Extension* (May 2006): 60.

4. Ibid., 63.

5. William Faloon, "No More Heart Attacks!" *Life Extension* (May 2009): 7–14.

6. P. M. Ridker, J. E. Buring, J. Shih, M. Matias, and C. H. Hennekens, "Prospective Study of C-reactive Protein and the Risk of Future Cardiovascular Events Among Apparently Healthy Women," *Circulation* 98 (1998): 731–733.

CHAPTER 3
DR. COLBERT'S TOP RISK FACTORS OF CARDIOVASCULAR DISEASE—AND HOW TO BEAT THEM WITH NUTRITION

1. M. Cesarone et al., "Improvement in Circulation and in Cardiovascular Risk Factors With a Proprietary Isotonic Bioflavonoid Formula OPC-3," *Journal of Angiology* 59 (2008): 408–414.

2. Frank F. Willems, Godfried H.J. Boers, Henk J. Blom, Wim R. M. Aengevaeren, and Freek W.A. Verheugt, "Pharmacokinetic Study on the Utilisation of 5-Methyltetrahydrofolate and Folic Acid in Patients With Coronary Artery Disease," *British Journal of Pharmacology* 141, no. 5 (March 2004): 825–830.

3. J. Danesh, S. Lewington, S. G. Thompson, et al., "Plasma Fibrinogen Level and the Risk of Major Cardiovascular Diseases and Nonvascular Mortality: An Individual Participant Meta-analysis," *Journal of the American Medical Association* 294, no. 14 (October 12, 2005): 1799–1809.

4. G. Coppola, M. Rizzo, M. G. Abrignani, et al., "Fibrinogen as a Predictor of Mortality After Acute Myocardial Infarction: A Forty-two Month Follow-up Study," *Italian Heart Journal* 6, no. 4 (April 2005): 315–322.

5. H. G. Langford, "Dietary Potassium and Hypertension: Epidemiological Data," *Annals of Internal Medicine* 98 (1990): 770–772.

6. Richard Hathaway, "How Aging Humans Can Slow and Reverse Atherosclerosis," *Life Extension* (March 2010): 42–43.

7. F. D. Kolodgie, A.P. Burke, K.S. Skorija, et al., "Lipoprotein-associated Phospholipase A2 Protein Expression in the Natural Progression of Human Coronary Atherosclerosis," *Arteriosclerosis, Thrombosis, and Vascular Biology* 26, no. 11 (November 2006): 2523–2529.

8. American Heart Association, "Alcohol, Wine and Cardiovascular Disease," http://www.americanheart.org/presenter.jhtml?identifier=4422 (accessed March 25, 2010).

10. G. B. Phillips, B. H. Pinkernell, T. Y. Jing, "Are Major Risk Factors for Myocardial Infarction the Major Predictors of Degree of Coronary Artery Disease?" *Metabolism* 53, no. 3 (March 2004): 324–329.

11. Edward Giovannucci, Yan Liu, Bruce W. Hollis, and Eric B. Rimm, "25-Hydroxyvitamin D and Risk of Myocardial Infarction in Men: A Prospective Study," *Archives of Internal Medicine* 168, no. 11 (2008): 1174–1180.

12. Johanna M. Geleijnse, Cees Vermeer, Diederick E. Grobee, et al., "Dietary Intake of Menaquinone Is Associated With a Reduced Risk of Coronary Heart Disease: The Rotterdam Study," *Journal of Nutrition* 134 (November 2004): 3100–3105.

13. R. E. Olson, "Vitamin K," in M. Shils, J. A. Olson, M. Shike, A. C. Ross, eds. *Modern Nutrition in Health and Disease*, 9th ed. (Baltimore: Williams & Wilkins, 1999), 363–380.

14. G. Ferland, "Vitamin K," in B. A. Bowman, R. M. Russell, eds., *Present Knowledge in Nutrition* 1, 9th ed. (Washington, DC: ILSI Press, 2006), 220–230.

15. William S. Harris, Kimberly J. Reid, Scott A. Sands, and John A. Spertus, "Blood Omega-3 and Trans Fatty Acids in Middle-Aged Acute Coronary Syndrome Patients," *American Journal of Cardiology* 99, no. 2 (January 15, 2007): 154–158.

16. M. Friedman, *Treating Type A Behavior and Your Heart* (New York: Ballantine Books, 1984), 33–43.

17. Stephen Sinatra and James Roberts, *Reverse Heart Disease Now: Stop Deadly Cardiovascular Plaque Before It's Too Late* (Hoboken, NJ: John Wiley & Sons, Inc., 2007), 46.

18. Jukka T. Salonen, Kristiina Nyyssonen, Heikki Korpela, et al., "High Stored Iron Levels Are Associated With Increased Risk of Myocardial Infarction in Eastern Finnish Men," *Circulation* 86, no. 3 (September 2002): 803–811.

CHAPTER 4
CHELATION THERAPY: HOPE FOR ENDING ANGINA

1. N. E. Clarke et al., "Treatment of Angina Pectoris with Dissodium Ethylene Diamine Tetraacetic Acid," *American Medical Journal of Medical Science* 232 (1956): 654.

2. Please note that there is some controversy surrounding the use of chelation therapy. For example, it is FDA approved for lead poisoning but not for atherosclerosis. If you'd like to look into this therapy further, I recommend the following book: Elmer Cranton, *Bypassing Bypass* (Troutdale, VA: Medex Publishers, 1990).

3. American Heart Association, "Questions and Answers About Chelation Therapy," http://www.americanheart.org/presenter .jhtml?identifier=3000843 (accessed March 31, 2010).

CHAPTER 5
NUTRITIONAL SUPPLEMENTS FOR CONGESTIVE HEART FAILURE AND ANGINA

1. Alexander Leaf, "On the Reanalysis of the GSSI-Prevenzione," *Circulation* 105 (2002): 1874–1875.

2. Christine M. Albert, Hannia Campos, Meir J. Stampfer, et al., "Blood Levels of Long-Chain n-3 Fatty Acids and the Risk of Sudden Death," *New England Journal of Medicine* 346, no. 15 (April 11, 2002): 1113–1118.

Don Colbert, MD, was born in Tupelo, Mississippi. He attended Oral Roberts School of Medicine in Tulsa, Oklahoma, where he received a bachelor of science degree in biology in addition to his degree in medicine. Dr. Colbert completed his internship and residency with Florida Hospital in Orlando, Florida. He is board certified in family practice and anti-aging medicine and has received extensive training in nutritional medicine.

If you would like more
information about natural and
divine healing, or information about
Divine Health nutritional products,
you may contact Dr. Colbert at:

DON COLBERT, MD

1908 Boothe Circle
Longwood, FL 32750
Telephone: 407-331-7007 (for ordering product only)
Dr. Colbert's Web site is
www.drcolbert.com.

Disclaimer: Dr. Colbert and the staff of Divine Health Wellness Center are prohibited from addressing a patient's medical condition by phone, facsimile, or e-mail. Please refer questions related to your medical condition to your own primary care physician.

Pick up these other great Bible Cure books by Don Colbert, MD: